TECHNICAL Terms frequently employed in Dancing.

à côté	...	means	...	to the side.
à gauche	...	„	...	to the left.
à droit	...	„	...	to the right.
dessus	...	„	...	over, or in front.
dessous	...	„	...	under, or rear.
avant	...	„	...	forward.
arrière	...	„	...	backward.
dedans	.	„	...	inwardly.
dehors	...	„	...	outwardly, or backward.
point	...	„		foot pointed with the weight of the body on the other foot.
supporting leg		„	..	the one on which the body is supported.
free leg	...	„	...	the one which is moving while the other supports the body.
pas	..	„	...	a complete step
temps	...	„	...	a syllable or portion of a step.
tempo	...	„	...	the time or the rhythm of the music.
vis-a-vis		„	...	facing each other.
révérence or salute			..	lady curtsey and gentleman bow simultaneously.

ABBREVIATIONS employed in the "Glossary."

R.—right.　　L.—left.　　F.—Foot.

H.—Hand.　　Pos.—Position.

Note.—The Editor is not responsible for the description of any step or movement given by the creators of the numerous dances in the Encyclopædia.

GLOSSARY.

A.B.C.—Alphabet.—POSITIONS.—The premier place in all study of the Art of Dancing must be given to the A.B.C. of the Art – the Positions, which form the fundamental principle of all dance movements.

There are five principal positions in six classes : (1) toe, (2) point, (3) ball, (4) sole, (5) heel, and (6) elevated positions.

The principal sole positions are :—

FIRST POSITION.—Place heels together and the toes well turned out, weight equally distributed on both feet and knees together.

SECOND POSITION.—Place the feet straight to the side in a line, with a space the length of the dancer's foot between them, the weight of the body on both feet. Should the feet be a greater distance from each other, they would then be said to be in a " double second " position.

THIRD POSITION.—Place the heel of one foot in the hollow of the other. If the heel of right foot is placed in the hollow of the left it will be " right foot to third front position "; if, however, the hollow of the right foot is placed against the heel of the left it will be " right foot to third position rear." In both cases it is the right foot moving ; should the left foot be making the movement, it would be " left foot to third front or rear." The weight is placed on both feet in the third position.

FOURTH POSITION.—Legs straight and one step forward is " fourth front position." The foot one step to the rear, at a distance of one foot, is fourth rear position.

FIFTH POSITION.—The legs and feet crossed so that the heel of one foot is directly opposite and touching the toe of the other. The feet would be exactly in front of each other and parallel. To practise this position it is as well to grasp a bar or chair. Owing to the formation of the foot, the right heel in the fifth position will touch the side of the left big toe, but the right small toe will touch the instep of the left foot.

The *first*, *third*, and *fifth* positions are called " *close positions*," the feet being together *close* and the weight on both.

The *second* and *fourth* positions are " *open positions*," the feet being *open* and apart.

TOE POSITION. In the positions already described if the extreme points of the toes are used it is the " *toe position*."

POINT POSITION.—If the toe only touches the ground with the weight on the other foot it is a " *point position*."

BALL POSITION.—If the ball or forward portion of the sole touches the ground it is a " *ball position*."

SOLE POSITION.—If the whole sole touches the ground it is a " *sole position*."

HEEL POSITION.—If the heel only touches the floor it is a " *heel position*."

ELEVATIONS OR FLOWING POSITIONS. - If a foot is raised entirely from the floor it will be an " *elevation* or *flowing position*." It may be a " *low elevation*," that is near the floor. " *Half-high elevation*," foot raised on a level with the calf of the other leg. " *High elevation*," foot raised as high as possible.

DIRECTION.--If the whole foot is on the ground it is in the " *horizontal direction* "; if the foot rests on the ball the direction is " *inclined* " or " *diagonal* "; if it is in the point position it is " *perpendicular* " or " *vertical* " ; and if on the heel it is " *upward* " or " *rebroussale* " direction (Rebroussale is derived from Fr. rebrousser, to turn up) from the pointing upward of the toes.

ELEVATIONS.—If the foot does not touch the floor, it is elevated. If raised a little from the floor to the side it is a "*second low elevation*." If raised forward it will be a "*fourth low front elevation*." If raised backward it will be a "*fourth low rear elevation*." If the foot is raised to the side, level with the other calf, it will be the "*second half-high elevation*"; if level with the hip it will be "*second high elevation*"; if the leg is raised forward or backward, it will be in the "*fourth front or rear elevation*."

While the body is being supported on one leg the other can balance in either "*stretched*," that is quite straight; "*half-stretched*," knee slightly bent; "*rounded*," bent slightly more and the leg from the knee to the toe in line with the other knee; "*half bended*," knees almost touching and leg high up rear; "*entirely bended*," the whole leg pushed backward and upward.

INTERMEDIATE POSITION.—Should the foot be placed in such a position that it is neither second nor fourth, but between the two, it is said to be in the "*intermediate position*." The foot can also be between the first and third, third and fifth, or second and fourth, &c.; these are all in the "*intermediate position*." A "*prolonged position*" is one in which the step is longer than the length of the foot, and is therefore exaggerated.

Abaisser (pronounced AH-BAY-SAY).—See Abaissements.

Abaissements (AH-BAISS-MAHN).—Lowerings. Two terms are employed for lowering—"*abaisser*," which signifies a lowering; and "*baisser*," putting down. To lift the right foot is "*lever* le pied droit," to put it down is "*baisser*." To raise oneself is s'elever — *i.e.*, to raise the heels from the floor; to assume the normal position, that is, to let the heels again touch the floor is *abaisser* or *s'abaisser*. Hence –

<blockquote>

Lever... ... To lift (the right or the left leg).
Baisser ... To put down (right or left leg).
s'Elever ... To raise oneself.
s'Abaisser ... To lower oneself. This must not be confused with plier.

</blockquote>

Academy of Dancing.—Founded by Louis XIV. in Paris. The Academicians were Florent du Desert, Prévot, Jean Renaud, Guillaume Renaud, Reynal, Guéru, d'Olivet, de Manthe, Jean Raynal, de Lorges, Picquet, Galant du Desert, and Jean de Grygny.

Accrochirisme (l'.)—Date 1503. Rhythm 3—4. A merry wrestle in which the dancers touch each other, then hook their arms round each other's body, revolving by élevés forward, backward and turning completely round. The overthrow of one or the other decided the victor.

Adage (l'.) (AH-DAHJH).—When the sublimity of the subject chosen is represented by postures, attitudes, play of the arms or countenance, in any position or in pirouetting.

À coin (AH-KWAHN).—To the corner.

À côté (AH-KO-TAY).—Sideways.

Adelienne (l'.) (AH-DEL-YEN).—1897. Created by Mdlle. Adelia da Silva Feixeira, Teacher of Dancing, Oporto. Composed to the music "Linger Longer Loo." During four bars introduction the dancers take their places. This dance then occupies 104 bars, followed by four bars finale to lead partners to seats.

Position. Gentleman stands at lady's side with her left hand in his right (*which will hereafter be termed the " Pas de Quatre position."*)

THE STEP. *Gentleman.* Bar 1.—(1) Point l.f. in front of r.f. (2) Repeat to the rear. (3) Repeat forward. (4) Raise the l.f. forward (en l'air), strongly bending r. knee.

Bar 2.—(1) Glide l.f. forward. (2) Glide r.f. forward. (3) Glide l.f. forward. (4) Pause.

Bars 3, 4,—Repeat 1, 2, commencing other foot, then release hands. *Lady* makes the same steps, but with the opposite foot.

Bars 5, 6.—*Gentleman.* (1) Glide l.f. to left slightly backward. (2) Pass point of r.f. close to l.f. outside and well crossed. (3) Pivot on the soles a three-quarter turn to left. (4) Pause. (5, 6) Glide l.f. to rear. (7, 8) Draw r.f. to l.f. facing each other and at a distance. *Lady* the same with opposite foot, pivoting to the right.

Bars 7, 8.—Both commencing r.f., approach each other with steps of Bars 1 and 2.

Bars 9 to 16.—Both join r. hands. Both commence l.f., and repeat bars 1 and 2 three times. The lady does a pirouette to l., and takes up the first position, and the whole is repeated five times, making 96 bars, then repeat bars 9 to 16 and 4 bars to lead lady to seat—108 bars. The lady holds her train with either or both hands when free. The gentleman places the free hand on the hip; when both hands are free, one rests on the hip and the other should be elevated.

À droit (AH-DROO-AH).—To the right.

À gauche (AH-GOHSH).—To the left.

Ailes de Pigeon (*les*) (I-DER-PIZHYON), *or pistolet.*—Some technical terms and names of dances are derived from the supposed resemblance of the step to some article or familiar movement; as *Cachuca*, which in Spain refers to anything pretty; *Pavane*, the graceful strut of a peacock. So, "ailes de pigeon" means literally "pigeon wings," and is so called from its supposed similarity to the "beat of the wings of a dove or pigeon.

The *simple* or in turning :—Bend l. leg and stretch the r. leg to 2nd position in the air (*2nd elevation*). In rising on the l. leg beat the r. calf against the l. (beneath the calf). Then beat the l. calf at the back of the right and fall on the r.f. with the l. leg outstretched in 2nd elevation. These two beats are performed with both feet off the floor and falling back on the r.f. This constitutes a "flap of the pigeons" to the right (or half wings); to complete the "ailes de pigeons" repeat commencing with other leg. These "ailes" are often executed 8 and 16 times according to the necessities of the dance. They are done in turning to the right or left; one turn for four half beats of the wings.

Ailes de Pigeon en terre.—On the ground. The same as the simple, but the feet must remain close to the ground and not elevated.

Ailes de Pigeon coupés.—L. leg to 2nd elevation. Rise on r. leg and beat l. calf against it, then beat r. calf against l. calf. Alight on l.f. and gliding r.f. to the right, glide l.f. to 3rd front (*assemblé*).

This step can also be done *en avant* (forward) and *en arriére* (backward).

Ailes de Pigeon berceau. (BER-SO). *Cradle step.*—Execute the simple wings once or three times, followed by a cradle step.

À la fin. (AH-LA-FANH).—At the finish.

Alberts.—A corruption of " The D'Alberts." A square dance.

Figure 1.	...	First figure of Quadrilles.
,, 2.	...	Second ,. of Caledonians.
,, 3.	...	Third ,, of Lancers.
,, 4.	...	Waltz Cotillon half through.
,, 5.	...	Fifth figure of Quadrilles (flirtation).

Allé. (*pas*) (PAH-ZAH-LAY). Walking step.—This step is generally called pas marché, but between walking and marching there is a great difference. Walking is to move easily, marching is a regulated step. In walking, the arms swing naturally, in marching they are carried in some prescribed manner. In walking, the stepping foot is put down to receive the weight of the body easily; in marching, the toe of the stepping foot is first placed on the ground. See Marché.

Allemande. (AHL-MAHND).—A dance in Switzerland and Germany about 1580. The music in 2-4 tempo was lively and gay. It was performed by the gentleman turning the lady under his arm and *vice versa*. In modern dances the *allemande* is done in the same manner, usually, however, it is the lady who pirouettes under the gentleman's upraised arm.

It has been asserted that the modern waltz owes its origin to the Allemande, but the fallacy of the argument will be apparent from the description of the allemande as danced in the reign of Henry IV. of France in 1590, and of Louis XV. in 1715. All the couples join hands in a circle and galop (*chasses*) round the room, first to the right, then to the left. Then, releasing hands, the gentlemen remain in their places while the ladies make a tour de bras (*or turn*) beneath the gentleman's arms, passing from one gentleman to the next as in the grande chaine of the modern Lancers; repeat the circle galop, each gentleman passing under the lady's arms; repeat the whole *ad lib*. In Switzerland the dance was varied by the gentleman turning the lady under one arm and then the other. There is not the remotest resemblance between this and the modern waltz. In 1565 (Charles IX) it was danced by a gentleman and two ladies. They went backwards and forwards, then the gentleman turned one lady under his arm, he, repeating the turn under her arm ; the dance recommenced, and he repeated the turns (allemande) with the other lady.

Allemande. (AHL-MAHND).—Dance composed by Théo. Lytle, 1897. Eight bars; tempo 2-4.

Position. Lady and gentleman, *vis-a-vis* (facing each other), left hands joined.

Gentleman, a polka step with left foot to the left. *Lady* simultaneously, polka step r.f. to the right.

Gentleman with r.f., *Lady* with l.f. a pas marché, diagonally forward.

Gentleman pivot a half-turn to left on the right sole and assemblé l.f. to 3rd rear. *Lady*, same step with opposite foot. Now change hands and repeat these two bars commencing with the other foot ; then waltz four bars and repeat the whole *ad lib*.

Alliance. (AHL-LE-AHNS).—Franco-Russian dance from Toulouse (1897). 16 bars, 2-4 and 16 bars 3-4 time.

Position as for Pas de Quatre. The gentleman's steps and lady's steps are similar, but the gentleman commences with the l.f. the lady with r.f.

THEORY FOR THE GENTLEMAN. 1st bar.—(1)   Glide l.f.
forward, obliquely to the left (2) pass r.f. in front of l.f., tapping the
point of the foot on the ground, the body bent to the right.

2nd bar.—Repeat first bar commencing r.f. and turning the
back a little.

3rd bar.—Repeat first bar exactly.

4th bar.—Glide r.f., bring l.f. up to it facing the lady, and,
releasing hands, salute.

Bars 5-8.—Repeat bars 1 to 4 ; finish bar 8 facing each other
(vis-a-vis) gentleman with hands on hips, lady with both hands
raising the dress.

Bar 9.—(1) Both glide r.f. to the right, (2) draw l.f. to r.f.

Bar 10.—(1) Both glide r.f. to the right, (2) Cross l f. in front
of r.f., tapping the toe on the floor, looking at each other.

Bars 11-12. - Repeat bars 9-10 with l.f., then join right hands
and perform a turn with the following step.

Bar 13.—(1) Glide r.f. in front of l.f. (2) Draw l.f. up to r.f.

Bar 14.—Repeat last bar with l.f.

Bars 15-16.—Repeat bars 13-14. The music then changes
to 3-4 tempo.

Bars 17-32.—Waltz 16 bars to Waltz music.

Repeat the whole *ad. lib.*

Alliance.—(Cronstadt, Toulon, 1890). 2-4 tempo.

For 2, 4, 6, or 8 couples placed in two parallel lines. Ladies in
French and gentlemen in Russian costume.

THEORY. *First Part.* 8 bars.—The two lines walk backward
and forward, tapping the sole on the floor, the gentlemen with
hands on hips, the ladies raising their dresses, answer by a
curtsey the salutations of the gentlemen.

Second Part. Four bars.—Both turn separately in their places,
the left hand on the hip, the right elevated above the head.

Third Part. Eight bars.—Promenade, and a tour de main
with partners.

Fourth Part. Four bars. - Two pas de basques, separately,
finishing with two pirouettes in place.

Fifth Part. Four bars.—Pas de basques holding hands,
finishing with a pirouette.

Sixth Part. Eight bars.—Promenade with pas de basques.

Seventh Part. 20 bars.—Repeat parts 1, 2, 3.

Eighth Part. Eight bars.—Jeté with r.f. then with l.f., followed
by three changements de talon (changes on the heels) moving
forward (2 bars). Repeat forward (2 bars). Repeat the whole
backward (4 bars).

Ninth Part. Eight bars.—*Fouetté* with r.f. forward, stretch
the right leg backward, three changements de jambe (changes of
the leg) and a Russian salute for the gentleman. The lady walks
round her partner with seven pointed dainty steps, then assemblé.
Repeat four times in all.

Tenth Part. Eight bars.—Promenade with chassés ouverts
(open chassés).

Eleventh Part. 20 bars.—Repeat parts 1, 2, 3.

Twelfth Part. Two bars.—Dégagé, fouetté, pointé, ballonné
with each foot.

Thirteenth Part. Two bars.—Pas de basque forward, brisé,
glissé backward twice.

Fourteenth Part. Eight bars.—Two pas marchés forward and one backward, and a Russian and Parisian salute (4 bars). Repeat (4 bars).

Fifteenth Part.—Place left arm round each other, the other elevated, turn in this position and finish with the hands of the gentlemen in those of the ladies.

Allonger (AH-LAWN-JHAY).—Stretching. Also *s'Allonger*, to stretch oneself. Article 119 of Zorn's " Grammar " states that " Stretching is a movement the reverse of bending, without which a new bend cannot be executed." *Redresser* is to make straight a bended leg. *Allonger* is to stretch out (see tendre). *Plier* is to bend the knees. Compare with " Abaisser."

Alphabet (AHL-FA-BET).—See A.B.C., also article " THEATRE."

Anapolies.—Ancient Greek dances in which wrestling was combined.

Anglaise (AHN-GLAYZ).—Theatrical. 2-4 time. 1, 2, 3, 4, or more dancers. In one figure there are four steps ; one to the right, one to the left, one forward, and one backward.

Début (entry). Promenade to the right during 8 bars : Sauter (hop) twice on l.f., making two *petits battements* with r.f. in front of l.f., jeté with r.f. forward ; repeat with other foot.

First Figure. Point to right and assemblé : point to left and assemblé : berceau (cradle-step, see *berceau*) forward eight times and assemblé : berceau eight times and assemblé.

Second Figure. Battement with the sole to the right and assemblé : petit battements (double ones) backward; berceau four times backward and assemblé.

Third Figure. Dégagé with r.f. to the right ; three changes of the heels, point the heels and assemblé—three times with r.f. Repeat with l.f. Rond de jambe with r.f., point toe and heel r.f. six times forward : foutté ; stretch out rounding the leg and assemblé : rond de jambe the l. to rear ; toe and heel six times to rear with l.f., fouetté before the r. leg; round forward the straight leg and assemblé.

Fourth Figure. Point five times with a change of heels ; point r. heel to 2nd position, then with the point in front of l.f., then to the side, then to rear four times with r.f. and assemblé. Repeat with l.f.

Ciseaux (se-so). *Forward.* Explanation of scissor-step. Place the toes together, heels open ; shut the heels and open the toes ; repeat eight times forward and assemblé.

Backward. Open the heels, close points : close heels and open the points—eight times backward and assemblé.

Fifth Figure, Ciseaux turning to right. *Analysis.* Open the heel of r.f. closing the toe of l.f., open the point of r.f. closing heel of l.f. and so on while turning, then assemblé ; repeat to left while turning. Point in 2-4 time with the r.f., then l.f., followed by a change of heels ; repeat four times forward and assemblé—repeat backward. Repeat from the " point," with l.f.

Sixth Figure. Ciseaux and grand écart (splits), rise, point forward and assemblé, four times forward : point backward and assemblé four times.

Seventh Figure. Point right 2nd position, repeat l.f., assemblé, three *trots de cheval* (pas cheval—horse steps) forward : berceau : frappé (tap) l.f., chassé r.f., frappé three times with double sole and berceau : three pas cheval, berceau and assemblé : (the pas cheval must be repeated backward as well as forward).

9

Eighth Figure. Point r.f. to 2nd position with toe and heel; fouetté forward and backward: three changes of the heels: repeat three times more to right and assemblé. Repeat the whole to the left. Ciseaux forward: six berceau: twice more forward, and assemblé. Repeat backward.

Ninth Figure. Sissonnes Anglaise to the right: berceau and assemblé: ailes de pigeon and berceau forward: (repeat five times forward) and assemblé: ailes de pigeon and berceau backward six times and assemblé.

Tenth Figure. Berceau turning to right and assemblé: repeat to left: point forward, ailes de pigeon and assemblé. Repeat backward.

Eleventh Figure. With r.f. battement with the sole in turning to the right and assemblé: repeat with l.f., battement the right sole forward, three chassés, frappé with the foot. Chassé with l., then with r., tapping with the feet three times forward and assemblé. Repeat backward.

Twelfth Figure. Open (échappé) to 2nd position and three changes of heels: repeat twice to right and assemblé terre à terre: berceau forward three times and assemblé. Repeat backward.

Thirteenth Figure. Three times ailes de pigeon and three changes of heels: ailes de pigeon coupé backward and forward: ailes de pigeon in place turning and assemblé.

Fourteenth Figure. Two écarts, three changes of heels: repeat this four times and assemblé: écart, double entrechat, écart, tour en l'air (turn in the air), repeat twice and assemblé for the finale. Promenade to the right as for the début; écart, entrechat, écart, entrechat, and final attitude.

Anglaise Militaire.—Either Solo or a number. 2-4 time. Début. Promenade to right and left.

First Figure. Tap right sole forward, fouetté r.f. in front of l.f., and a scissor-step with l.f. Repeat with l.f. Tap sole to rear to finish.

Second Figure. Double beat right sole forward, beat r.f. to right, three fouettés, tap with foot and fouetté. Repeat with l.f. Double beat the sole to rear to finish the figure.

Third Figure. Pas cheval forward, dégagé with r.f,, entrechat and three points. Repeat with l.f. and finish with pas cheval to rear.

Fourth Figure. Ciseaux forward, demi-ciseaux, three changes of the feet to the right; semi-diseaux and three changes of the feet to left; finish with ciseaux to rear.

Fifth Figure. Beat three times with the sole in walking forward: ciseaux in turning to the right; ciseaux turning to left. Beat three times with the sole going backward.

Sixth Figure. Chassé-croisé, two fouettés, demi-ailes de pigeon forward, two points, assemblé and three changes of the feet to the right. Repeat to the left. Finish with chassé-croisé, two fouettés and demi-ailes de pigeon to the rear.

Seventh Figure Bourrée forward, three changes, three points, assemblé on the points, jumping twice on r.f. Repeat l.f. Finish with Bourrée, to rear and three changement de jambes.

Eighth Figure. Triolet forward, ballonné to right and left. Triolet to rear.

Ninth Figure. Dégagé forward, half terre-à-terre, ciseaux, beat with sole, triolet turning to right. Repeat with l.f. Finish with échappé, demi-terre-à-terre, ciseaux and tap the sole.

Tenth Figure. Two points, demi-rond-de-jambe, demi-ailes de pigeon forward and fouetté, turning to right. Repeat with l.f. Finish with two points, demi-rond-de-jambe and demi-ailes de pigeon to rear.

Eleventh Figure. Points, demi-ciseaux forward, ballonné, triolet to the right. Repeat to left. Finish with points and demi-ciseaux to rear.

Twelfth Figure. Terre-à-terre forward, dégagé, half terre-à-terre, demi-ciseaux, assemblé forward, ciseaux, three changement de jambe (changes of the legs) to the right. Repeat left. Terre-à-terre to the rear.

Thirteenth Figure. Demi-rond-de-jambe, run forward, point, coupé to the right, ciseaux, changement de pied (foot) to the left, ailes de pigeon coupé to rear. Finale. Promenade as at début to right and left (start on the points and lower yourself) écart and entrechat.

Anglicane (l') (LAHN-GLEE-KANE).—Date 1530, Henry VIII. of England. 2-4 time. Eight steps to four bars. Gentleman's step. Glide l.f. to left. Coupé r.f. dessous (below). Describe a demi-rond (half-cirele) en l'air (in the air) with l.f.; jeté with l.f. and assemblé (2 bars). Repeat with r.f. (2 bars.) Tombé in 3-time twice to each side. The Gentleman and lady commence with joined hands and opposite feet. They release hands for the tombés (falls).

Angrismene (l') or the *Fâchée* (FAH-SHAY).—Greek Pantomime Dance for a couple, 1821. 3-4 time. Placed next his partner, in step and gesture the man developes all the passion of love. He simulates strangulation with a handkerchief because he disbelieves in her love. She runs to him, cuts away the handkerchief and restores him, deploring and upbraiding him for his severity. He recovers and they vow eternal fidelity. They dance face to face, expressing their mutual sentiments by facial expression, gesture and movements of the body and legs. They pirouette and dance a duet, the man finishing on his knees at his partner's feet.

Aplomb (AH-PLON).—With assurance. To alight neatly and with assurance on the feet after any step.

Apotheosis.—Final Tableau. The artistic combination of the scene-painter, the decoration of the architecture, the costumier, the harmony of colours, and the sparkling grouping of the dancers. The dancers study their attitudes, electricity plays its part by throwing fires of all colours on the human throng. The subjects vary infinitely and depend mainly on the idea intended to be conveyed: a person recovered, be it king or queen, surrounded by their suite, the attitudes varying according to taste; a representation of an engagement in war; a king with his staff officers or his seraglio; a queen with her ladies-in-waiting, etc., etc. Facts and historical subjects can be represented, personages arrayed in costumes and accessories, arms, flowers, etc; everything, indeed, which can give an impression, realistic or ideal, of the author's thought. The attitudes of the dancers are innumerable. The subjects are pourtrayed in the painting of the sky, in the trees, the flowers, the fields, the clouds, even space suspended by a thread, in the sun, in jewels, in arms, in the field of battle, etc. It is the finale of the ballet or play: it is a god which should impress on the audience the general idea of the play.

Arabesque (AH-RA-BESK).—The position of the body in attitudes. Groups of dancers, male or female, or both, entwined by various properties such as scarves, flowers, rings. ribbons, hoops, garlands, etc. Sometimes the dancers, from their groupings and attitudes, represent antique bas-reliefs, or the painting on a great scale of the ideal or passion of some myth, god or person. The best arabesques and attitudes can be studied from the antique Grecian and Roman marbles.

Arcadian.—By R. M. Crompton (1897). Music by Morley. Eight measures in 3-4 Mazurka tempo. The dance, for couples, is composed of a series of eight bars repeated.

Archimime (ARSH-E-MEEM).—Tempo 2-4. A dance in imitation of the life of a person being taken to the cemetery, the funeral pyre or the gallows. The Romans danced it in the presence of the criminal or sufferer, performing such steps, gestures and attitudes as would convey to him the good and bad actions of his lifetime.

Argentine Tango.—*See* Tango.

Arlequine (ARL-KAN).—Theatrical. For couples vis-a-vis. Tempo 2-4. 1st step, dance with rond de jambe turning. 2nd step, tombè to the side, bending twice to the right and twice to the left. 3rd step, Pirouette to left, écart and entrechat three times; this is done in a square. 4th step, casse-cou in place, one bar. 5th step, contretemps to left and three tirés (drawing steps) and entrechat; this is done in a square. 6th step, bourrée in place and four tirés; this is done to right and left. 7th step, chassé ouvert (open) on all four sides. 8th step, cross to one side with jetés, spreading out the arms to form a cross to the left : twice. 9th movement, wag the head keeping arms still. 10th step, glissade to right, jeté, bourrée: repeat the glissade, jeté, bourrée to face each other: twice. 11th step, jeté-en tournant (in turning), écart and entreehat on four sides. 12th step, jeté-en-tournant to right, three tirés, entrechat and pirouette-en-l'air—on four sides. 13th step, bourrée forward, chassé, jeté, entrechat, stretch out the leg and dip from the hips ; jeté backward, entrechat and pirouette. Repeat to return to place.

Arlequine de Concert.—Tempo 2-4. Solo or duet. 1st, wave the wand, tap with it three times and entrechat. 2nd, three piqués (toe and heel) one change of the feet and entrechat. 3rd, contretemps, brisé and entrechat. 4th, demi-ciseaux (half scissor step), glissade and brisé. 5th, échappé, emboité, entrechat to rear, ballonné and entrechat. 6th, terre-à-terre, déboité to rear and ailes de pigeon-coupés. 7th, two piqués with each leg, tombé on each leg, bourée and seven brisés. 8th, Seven chassés backward, pirouette : four times. 9th, échappé, two fouettés, tombé, bourée, brisé, entrechat. 10th, wave the wand gracefully. 11th, écart, entrechat, changement, entrechat. 12th, three dégagés, changement, entrechat and promenade.

Arlesienne.—(1898). Danced by the children of Symphorien near Tours. 2-4 tempo. The children, in couples, facing each other, shod in sabots. (1) they take arms and advance, two taps of the sabot to the vis-a-vis (2 bars). Repeat backward, tap sabot to the lady and release arms (2 bars). Promenade. smiling at vis-a-vis in passing (8 bars). Boy clasps girl and the other hand on the hip. Polka piquée (toe and heel polka) round in place (8 bars). (4)

repeat 1. (5) promenade, tapping the sabots to accompany the music (8 bars). (6) ballonné. turning singly in place (4 bars). (7) repeat 1. (8) boy, polka-sautés round his partner ; girl repeat (8 bars), (9) boys and girls, polka forward, boys smile mockingly at vis-a-vis. (10) girls, with a menacing air, make boys escape to their partners (4 bars). All retire with polka and taps of the sabots (8 bars). Boys kneel on r. knee in attitude with their partners.

Arnaoute (AHR-NOOT).—Martial dance of the Greeks, 1700. Tempo 2-4. Gentlemen armed with sticks, ladies with whips. One couple agitates these, at the same time moving forward running, jumping and galloping. The other couples follow with hands interlaced, imitating the movements and gestures of the first couple. In ancient times the Greeks went to war led by this dance ; the success of the battle was supposed to depend on the couples who executed the dance, and conducting the army to glory or to death.

Arondi (AH-RON-DEE).—A rounded arm. The third degree of the bended arm. *See* Bras.

Arrêt, commonly known as "pas d'arrêt" (PAH-DAHR-RAY).—A checked or half-finished step—a pause with one leg suspended or raised, as in the Tango and Maxixe.

Arriére en (AH-REE-AIR).—To retire, as in square dances. Arrière rear. *See* Avant.

Assemblé (AH-SAHM-BLAY).—To bring together. Bringing the feet from an open to a close position in one tempo, or from one close position to another. The foot can be placed in *front* in the 1st, 3rd, or 5th position ; termed *assemblé dessus* ; if to the *rear* it is termed *assemblé dessous*. Continuous pas assemblés must be made with alternate feet.

Astronomique.—Egyptian dance. 600 B.C. Said to have been invented by Pythagoras The dancers were arranged in series of eight couples, from which one became detatched. All moved about with pas glissés and represented the course of the stars and the harmony of their'movements, by well-regulated figures, arranged in advance.

Attitude.—Harmonic position of the whole body in dancing or in repose. The feet and arms must assume the most graceful position, and harmonize with the subject the dance represents. The dancer maintains this position on one or both feet and facing in any direction. Only the most beautiful ideals, and not burlesques, should be represented. Strenuous and unceasing practice is necessary to attain the movements for the *opposition* of the arms, the body, the head and the legs to maintain easy and graceful attitudes. *See* Arabesque.

Auvergnate (O-VERN-YAHT). - Tempo 3-4. Date 1519, under Catherine de Medicis, who danced it. As many couples as desire may join ; they are placed in two parallel lines, each couple having its vis-a-vis, with whom they danced. The step is a kind of Pas-de Valse in 2-4 tempo, tapping the feet in time to the music. All the couples advance and retire agitating the arms, tapping the feet and changing places. Gentlemen only, repeat this, then ladies. Back to places. Turn round each other with tour-de main. Repeat all. Finale—clasp each other and dance round the room.

13

Avant (AH-VAHN).—Forward, or in front. *En avant*, to advance (as in Square dances).

Avant-*un, deux, trois, quatre, six, huit*.—One, two, three, four, six, or eight advance. Employed in the various Quadrilles. The step usually consists of three pas marchés and an assemblé.

Avant-un, is an advance solo, as in 2nd figure of Caledonians.

Avant-deux, two advance. This may be performed by a gentleman and his partner or a gentleman and his vis-a-vis.

Avant-trois, three advance; as in 4th figure of Quadrilles.

Avant-quatre, four advance. Two couples vis-a-vis advance.

Avant-six, six advance. *Example:*—First and second couples advance to side couples (*avant-quatre*), and, leaving the lady there, the gentlemen retire alone. The two sides will now each consist of three dancers, if they advance they will perform *avant-six*.

Avant-huit, eight advance, either in two lines or circle; as in 5th figure of Lancers, or Grand Circle.

À vos Places (AH-VO-PLAHS.) " Regain your places."

B

Baissé (BAIS-SAY).—A lowering time. *See* Abaissements.

Baisser (BAIS-SAY).—" Letting down " the raised limb.

Balancé (BAH-LAHN-SAY). With this expression is always implied the conception of remaining in place. (1) glide r.f. to 2nd or 4th position, dégagé; (2) glide l.f. to 3rd position, front or rear, and lightly raise the heels and let them down again. This movement is sometimes called " setting." It may be done à coté, en avant, en arriére, or en tournant.

Balancez.—Balancé is the noun or name of the movement. Balancez is the verb or action ; in this sense, " balancez " means " perform a balancé." *Se-balancer* is to rock oneself. When this movement was introduced into the first figure of the Quadrille, the dancers rocked from one foot to the other. The modern name for it is " Balancé a votre dame," better known as " setting to partners." and many teachers adhere to " balancé." To dance it. Preparation :— Face partners (1, 2, 3), commencing with r f., walk three ordinary steps sideways to the right, away from partner. (4) assemblé l.f to 3rd front. (5, 6, 7) commencing with l.f. return to places with three ordinary steps sideways to the left. (8) assemblé r.f. to 3rd rear. The whole occupies four bars of music.

Balancé-de-Menuet.—*See* Menuet.

Balancé-en-ligne (BAH-LAHN-SAY AHN-LEEN).—Balancé step, or " setting-in-line," as in 3rd figure of Quadrille.

Balayage (*pas de*) (BAH-LAH-YAHJH).—From belayer, to sweep. Imitate with one foot the sweep of a broom (coup de balai), rubbing the floor with the point of the foot, right to left or left to right, giving the movement of va-et-vient (come and go).

Ballerine (BAH-LER-REEN).—Dance. 3-4 tempo. Position as for Pas de Quatre. Left hands joined, gentleman's right arm round lady's waist. Gentleman commences with l.f., lady with r.f. The step is a pas marché on the sole, followed immediately by lowering the heel. The Dance. (1, 2, 3, 4) four pas marchés as described. (5) glide l.f. forward and draw point of l.f. to point of r.f., r. knee open, and slighty incline the head, and torso to the right. (6) temps d'arrêt, (pause) (2 bars). Repeat reversed (2 bars). Repeat first 2 bars. Pas-de-ballerine sideways, lady to left, gentleman to right, with r. hand on hips, still retaining l. hands. At the third beat the lady should incline head and bust to the left. The gentleman is now facing forward and the lady backward (2 bars). Gentlemen alone make a half turn to the left and place r. arm round partner. Both are now facing the other way ; repeat the whole in the opposite direction, followed by eight bars waltz or polka-lente in 3-4 time. The dance can be executed à droit, à gauche, en avant, en arrière, or en tournant.

Ballet (BAH-LAY).—A chorus of dancers, who, by action, pourtray human sentiments and passions. Supposed to have been invented by the ancient Egyptians The dancing in ballets should be part of the story. The principal is called "première ballerino" or "première danseuse."

Ballet d'Action (BAH-LAY DAHK-TZE-ON). Sometimes termed "**Danse d'Action.**" - Ordinary ballet or play where gesture and dancing replaces dialogue. A "divertissement" is a scene in a ballet.

Ballet Chinois (BAH-LAY SHEEN-WAH.—Tempo 2-4. From two to fifty dancers. 1st step, pas-russe-en-tournant (*Russian step turning*). 2nd step, Ballonné, to front and to rear. 3rd step, fouetté-en-tournant. 4th step, two piqués, three changement-de-pieds. 5th step, demi-rond de jambe, two emboités. écart. 6th step, three times écart, demi-tour with ailes-de-pigeon. 7th step, jeté to right and left, three changement-de-pieds backward and three fouettés with each foot.

Ballet Cosaque (BAH-LAY KOS-SAHK).—Tempo 2-4. For as many as can be placed in two parallel lines. Introduction :—Promenade with pas russe. Each of the following steps should be concluded with a *pas finale*, which, however, may be omitted. *Theory of pas finale.* Stretch r. leg to right side ; jump on the two feet to the left side , slide r.f. to right side ; assemblé l.f. to rear ; two taps of the sole and point of the r.f. to the side and assemblé ; repeat taps with l.f.

1st step, sissonnes forward with r.f., then l.f. and pas finale ; repeat to rear. 2nd step, sissonnes with l.f., same with r.f., spring open and close twice ; three changements-de-pieds. Repeat with r.f. 3rd step, chassés ouvert (open) to the right ; three grands battements with l.f., and assemblé to rear. Repeat the other way. 4th step, three pas russe forward, brisés doublés, écart, entrechat, two pirouettes volantes (flying) and two beats of ailes de pigeon-coupé. Repeat. 5th step, two battements forward with r.f., assemblé and grand battement with l.f. ; three sissonnes to rear and assemblé. Repeat. 6th step, pas cheval to the right, grands battements with l.f., assemblé and five ailes de pigeon. Repeat to left, then to right and to the rear. 7th step, four Emboités forward, écart, entrechat, two ailes de pigeon-coupés to the rear. Repeat forward. 8th step, three écarts, three changements de pieds, three grand battements with r. leg and three changements; repeat battements with l. leg and three changements. 9th step, écart chinois (Chinese), assemblé, three changements, ; repeat; grand écart, one tiré to right, heels together. grand écart, entrechat. 10th step, promenade round the stage; then to finish, grand battement with r. leg to side and assemblé; repeat with l, ; contretemps and assemblé; grand battement with l. then r., contretemps and assemblé; two ailes de pigeon to rear, same in place, same forward, écart, entrechat, two ailes de pigeon forward, écart and entrechat.

Ballet for 10 Young Ladies.—Tempo 3-4. All dressed in white; the four tallest with soft clinging scarves four yards long, tightly wrapped round the waist. These are numbered 1 ,2, 3, 4 ; the others without scarves 5, 6, 7, 8 ; and two little girls (10 in all).

Figure 1.   Entry by Promenade in couples in following manner—Pas de Valse forward (1 bar); repeat, turning the back to the line of direction (1 bar). Changement de mains (change hands) and pas de valse backward (1 bar), pas de valse turning to face line of direction (1 bar), and repeat to take positions for the next figure.

Figure 2.   Dance the Valse Menuet by Crompton.

Figure 3.   Nos. 5, 6, 7, 8 take the ends of the scarves of 1, 2, 3, 4 ; and 1, 2, 3, 4 solo valse to unroll them (8 bars). Simultaneously 5, 6, 7, 8 follow, rolling themselves in the scarves. 1, 2, 3, 4 return rolling up scarves, 5, 6, 7, 8, meanwhile unrolling (8 bars). Unroll again, allowing the scarves to fall so that the first just touches the ground, the second a little higher, and the others in the same proportion (8 bars). The two little girls who were in the background now run on beside each other.

Figure 4.   The children solo waltz separately between and round the elder girls. Meeting in the centre they link right arms and make one and a half turns.

Figure 5.   The eight ladies arrange the scarves on the floor in a star, throwing them high in the air four times, the children alone dancing solo beneath and outside each time the scarves go up or down.

Figure 6.   The eight ladies do a complete turn with pas de valse, the children taking places, one at the back, the other in front.

Figure 7.   The ladies arrange the scarves in four lines, throwing them in the air, the children meanwhile dance beneath them and pirouetting as the scarves fall. Repeat until the children arrive in the centre a second time.

Figure 8.   The eight ladies arrange the scarves in a square with the children in the centre.

Figure 9.   The children dance a duet—a Gavotte, Menuet, Bolero or any other dance.

Figure 10.   1, 2, 3, 4 pas de valse to opposite line, rolling up scarves: they fall into couples and mutually (in dancing) roll them- selves up in the scarves.

Finale.   Each couple waltz round rolled up in a scarf, and make an effective tableau.

Ballet Pantomime.—Same as ballet d'action, but more often applied to the ballets seen in Christmas pantomime as distinct from " grand ballets."

Ballet Zingari.—For three boys and three girls. During eight bars introduction the three couples dance on, holding hands and in one line. They release hands, boys salute, girls curtsey. Approach partners, boy taking girl's hand. Centre couple (No. 1) retire two steps; the two other couples face each other; the couple on the right (No. 2) the other on the left (No. 3) forming a triangle. All this in eight bars introduction.

Figure 1. Number 1 approach centre with three small pas marchés, release hands and turn backs to each other. All salute. Couples 2 and 3 raise arms (2 bars), girl 1 pass beneath arm of couple 2, boy 1 beneath arms of couple 3, and both return to places with four pas marchés (2 bars). All boys take girls' r. hands in theirs and turn them beneath right arms (allemande), bow and curtsey (2 bars), change to left hands, allemande and salute as before (2 bars).

Figure 2. Couples 2 and 3 advance and retire, while they are retiring couple 1 advance. Boys advance to centre, face partners and bow and curtsey (4 bars). Boys kneel on one knee and give hands to partners. Girls pass to the right, round partners with tour de mains. They release hands and curtsey, inviting partners to rise (4 bars).

Figure 3. Boys join left hands in the centre and make a complete tour de moulinet with two polka and four pas marchés (4 bars). Release hands and perform the same steps, moving round their partners (4 bars).

Finale. Girls' left hands in boys' right. All, two polka steps and four pas marchés, following each other in couples round the circle (4 bars). Repeat the steps, going round in place (4 bars), Repeat, going round the circle (4 bars). Form a circle and repeat (4 bars). Boys kneel on r. knee, hands uplifted; girls remain in attitude. Boys rise, all salute and retire in couples.

Ballonné, *pas*, or BALLON (BAH-LONNAY) *Ball-step.*—The step is so called from the circular appearance of the free leg, which moves like stepping over as a ball. It can be made in any direction, but the most usual is sideways. If the circular movement is made without dégagé it is called *temps ballonné*. Stand in r. 5th position forward. (1) During a hop on l.f. the r. leg is carried in a circular line to 2nd position and dégagé. (2) Glide l.f. to 5th rear. If the next step is in the same direction, there is a dégagé on l.f., so that the r.f. may become free, but if the steps are to be made alternately, the dégagé is omitted and the movements can be repeated to the left.

Ballonné en sautant (SO-TAHN).—Sautant is jumping. In lightly jumping twice on l.f. (imitating the elastic fall and rebound of an air-ball) make two petits battements with r.f. in front of l.f., then dégagé on r.f. forward and draw l.f. to 5th rear (1 bar).

Ballonné retrograde.—A combination of steps of four measures. 1st Measure, pas ballonné to the right. 2nd Measure (1), l.f. to 2nd position; (2) glide r. toe to 5th forward, and the heel is then audibly put down while the l.f. is raised; (3) l.f. to 2nd position. 3rd Measure (1), r.f. to 2nd with dégagé; (2, 3) make a whole turn on r. toe or heel, by which l.f. is first raised to 2nd elevation, then to 5th rear with dégagé. 4th Measure (1), r.f. frappé into 5th rear, dégagé; (2) pause; (3) ballonné is begun as a preparation for the next step.

Ballon (BAHL-LON).—When a dancer's movements are graceful and elastic like a bounding ball.

17

Balloté or **Ballottés** (BAH-LOTTAY).—To toss about. When the feet are crossed alternately one before or behind the other. Two coupés following each other is a good example of "*pas ballotté.*" The "English Sailor Step" (*Pas de Matelot Anglais*) is a familiar example of the *triple pas ballotté* with a whip time (*temps fouetté*) into the forward elevation. "*Ballotté* is a step produced by swinging and alternate outward and inward throwing of the leg—strictly speaking, consisting of a coupé dessus and dessous—in two beats uniformly accented, and can be executed in place or en tournant."—KLEMM.

Ballottée.—(Danse). Common time. Couples place themselves as for pas de quatre. Lady's step; gentleman's the same, but with other foot. Glissade r.f. to 4th; chassé l.f.; glissade r.f. to 4th; l.f. to 4th forward elevation—facing each other (1 bar). Repeat with other foot, turning the back (1 bar). Back-to-back, make four balancés, imitating waves, and executing pas ballottés (2 bars). In waltz position they do eight very quick pivots on alternate feet (4 bars). Return to first part and repeat *ad lib.*

Bal Masqués.—The invention of the masqués dates back to the ancient Greeks, who employed them for theatrical performances. The idea of performers rendering themselves unrecognisable, for the sake of diversion, certainly dates from antiquity. In country villages, some of the villagers possess costumes which have been handed down during many past generations, and at certain seasons of the year, they are donned to perplex their neighbours in a house to house visitation. During carnivals, bals masqués and travesties have formed part of the festivities. In history, they are mentioned as having been the fashion at Court in the 14th century. After an accident at a Bal Masqué, the madness of Charles VI. of France increased. The Edict of November 26th, 1535, forbidding the manufacture and wearing of masks, had the effect of making them more popular, definitely and permanently establishing them as part of the pastimes of the people. The attraction of such forbidden fruit served but to whet the appetite of the pleasure-seeker, and, up to the time of the Revolution, the mask was used in times of rejoicing to hide the identity of the wearer. In modern times, the dress at a bal masqué is made to differ as much as possible from the costume of the period and the country. Their variety is infinite; classical, ancient, historical, mythical, comic, serious, and imaginative. Dominoes (the long loose Italian silk mantles with removable hoods) are also used as a general disguise. The security of a rigorous incognito adds much to the pleasure and piquancy of the ball. The liberty is greater, but within the limits of good taste. Sometimes the costume is restricted to that of certain countries; the characters depicted by chosen authors, such as Shakespere, Dickens, Dumas, etc.; periods of time or history; subjects of artists; the use of special material such as calico, etc. Originality is the first consideration, beauty even being sacrificed for the sake of novelty.

Barbette (LA).—1730. Tempo 2-4. Danced in couples by pas glissés, chassés and tournés in all directions; then the men kneel while the women pretend to pass a blade or a razor over them.

Barn Dance.—Imported from America; was originally danced in England to the music of Meyer Lutz's "Pas de Quatre," by which name the dance was for some time known. It is now almost obsolete. The gentleman takes his partner's left hand in his right and he beginning with l.f., she with r.f. execute a polka step forward (count 3), he raises r.f. forward, she l.f. forward (count 4); repeat with the other foot (count 4); repeat the whole (count 8), and four waltz movements. The whole is repeated *ad lib*. Another way: in common time. Three pas marchés and a pas sauté, four times, instead of the polka step.

Basque, Pas de (PAH-DER-BAHSK).—Sometimes called Pas Russe, and often mispronounced " Pas de pah " and " Pas ba."

The Basque people, who supply the origin of the name of this step, are those who dwell on the Bay of Biscay, that is N.W. of Spain and S.W. of France, close to the Pyrenees. The step plays an important rôle in Spanish dances, such as Cachucha, Bolero, Gitana, &c. The Pas de Basque consists of a suite of three steps in either 2-4 or 3-4 tempo; a half, a whole, and a half step. The accent can be made on either the first or second temps. When danced in common time there is either a pause or a hop for the fourth beat. *Forward*, from r.f. in 5th front position, bend slightly and round r.f. to second dégagé (count 1); glide l.f. through 1st, 3rd, and 5th positions into 4th forward dégagé, which in practice is an inward demi-rond de jambe en terre (count 2); assemblé r.f. to 3rd or 5th rear (count 3). Another pas de basque can now follow commencing with l.f. *Backward*, stand as in commencing the forward step. Jeté with l.f. to 2nd position (1); glide r.f. to 4th rear dégagé (2); l.f. to 5th front (3). *In place*, the 2nd step must go to 2nd position; the other steps the same as before. *En tournant*; as a rule the line of turning is backward; jeté r.f. sideways and backward to 4th rear with a simultaneous pivot of a half-circle on l.f. (1); l.f. is thrown over r.f., turning another half-circle (2); assemblé r.f. to 5th rear (3). Another description. With an outward circular movement of r. leg, glide forward or sideways on r.f., immediately raising l.f. to 4th forward elevation (1). Glide l.f. to 4th forward dégagé (2). Close r.f. to 3rd or 5th dégagé (3).

Battements (BAHT-MAHN).—Literally, beatings; derived from the word battre, to beat. If a foot is strongly pushed, beaten or knocked against the other it is a *battement*. There are two classes: GRAND BATTEMENTS, or high beatings, and PETITS BATTEMENTS, or low beatings; they may be made in all directions. GRANDS BATTEMENTS *en avant* : Stand in 3rd position. Throw the right leg out forward as high as possible, and let it fall back to the same close position from which it started. In grands battements the toes leave the floor last in lifting the leg and touch the floor first in lowering, the body must be held firmly on the supporting leg without swaying. GRANDS BATTEMENTS *de côte* : In the same manner the leg can be elevated sideways instead of forwards, and let it fall back beating the other foot as before. GRANDS BATTEMENTS *en arriére* : The leg is elevated to the rear and let fall. PETITS BATTEMENTS *(small beatings)*: These should be done only *de côté (sideward)*. Stretch one leg in second point position and quickly back to 5th position, either *dessus* or *dessous*. The active foot constantly moves from 2nd to 5th position. BATTEMENTS CROISÉS CHANGÉS *(changed crossed beatings)*: when the free foot beats the supporting foot alternately front and rear. Grands and petits battements are excellent practice for producing brilliancy in dancing.

BATTEMENTS VOLÉ; (1) coupé; (2) échappé; (3) battement in the air falling in 5th forward position. BATTEMENT RETOMBÉ : The l.f. being in 2nd elevation, lower it to 5th forward, and, in making a jump to the right, the l. strikes the r. and returns to 2nd elevation; this can be repeated *ad lib.* BATTEMENT DE SEMELLE, *battement of the sole* : Simple and forward on the floor. For Jigs, etc. From 3rd position raise r. knee and tap r. toe on the ground, stretch the leg out quickly forward in such a manner that in letting the foot return to the 3rd position, the sole again strikes the floor.

Battre (BAHTR).—To beat; the origin of the word "battement" (a beat). To distinctly beat or touch the supporting foot or leg with the other. The free leg goes from an open to a closed position, striking against the sole, heel, toe, calf or whole leg, either once, twice or more times, either dessus or dessous or alternately. (*See* Battu).

Battu (BAHTU).—Beaten. (*See* Battre). If the foot beats in front once against the other it is termed "*battu simple dessus.*" One beat to the rear "*battu simple dessous.*" Two beats, one in front and one to the rear "*battu alternatif.*" They can be executed in all positions, and in all choreographic steps.

Battu, Pas (PAH BAH-TU).—The full title should be "*pas battu latéral.*" It is also known by the names PAS POLONAISE and COUP DE TALON (knocking with the heels). If when knocking the heels together the legs are held well outward, the knock is liable to come against the ankle of the other foot, which is painful. The feet therefore are held almost parallel, and the step can be called "*pas battu parallel.*" The word latéral indicates that the step should be made sideways. For shortness the term "pas battu" is used. Example : The l.f. being raised in 2nd elevation, (temps 1), knock l. heel against the r. during a light hop on the r.f. (temps 2), step on l.f. to 2nd position, (temps 3), assemblé r.f. in 1st position and immediately raise l.f. ready for the next step. Another example : Bend r. knee, raise yourself, tapping l. calf against the r. tibia (shin-bone), with the calves nearly together, either to the side, forward, to the rear, or in turning in the air, according to the necessities of the dance. The battus can be doubled or tripled (in passing and en battant), forward, rear, falling on one foot, or tombé assemblé (falling-assemblé).

Bébé Biarritz (BAY-BAY BE-AH-RITS).—Baby Polka. Tempo 2-4. The boys and girls are arranged in the centre of the room in two lines, boys facing the girls, hands on the hips. Boys retire and girls advance with eight polka steps (8 bars.) Turn partners with r. hands, repeat with l. (8 bars). Tap three times with r.f., then three with l.f. (2 bars). Tap r. hands three times, then l. hands three times (2 bars). Lift r. hands and point with first finger, teasing partner, and do a turn in place with l.f. and come back to position again (4 bars). Repeat the whole twice and finish with Polka or Galop.

Berceau (**Pas**) (PAH BERSO).—(*Cradle Step*). Also BERCEUSE, a lullaby or rocker. So-called from its resemblance to the rocking of a cradle. It is executed with alternate foot, forward, backward, in place or turning ; the arms folded in front level with the shoulder or hands resting on hips. It is the "rocking step" in hornpipes, reels, jigs, &c. Example : From 3rd position stretch l.f. to 2nd elevation, then pass it in front of the right, the left calf touching the right tibia, and the point of the l.f. 5 centimetres (1·9685 inches or nearly two inches) from the point of the r.f. In this position move or rock the two legs together to the right side, then to left, then to right, then stretch the right to second elevation. Repeat these berceau movements with right foot. The body must not move, only the legs sway right and left, with open knees slightly bent, with elasticity and quickly. During the three swaying movements the feet do not change places. BERCEAU EN AVANT (*advancing*) : Three movements must be made on the points and advancing with each movement ; this needs power which can be acquired with practice. DEMI-BERCEAU is done with one foot without change, that is, another rocking movement is substituted for the elevation in the fourth beat. BERCEAU EN ARRIÈRE (backward) is made by passing the foot to the rear instead of in front on the first beat and moving backward during the rocking motion. BERCEAU EN TOURNANT (in turning) to right or left can be performed by rocking round in a circle to right or left. BERCEAU SUR LES POINTES are executed on the toes in all directions as already explained and are done like the sweep of a broom—va-et-vient, *i.e.*, going and coming—imitating the motion of a cradle ; they are the most beautiful of the berceau steps, and when the dancer excels in them the feet seem not to touch the ground. Another example : Stand l.f. in 2nd pos. elevation. (1) Throw l.f. over r.f. with dégagé, simultaneously raise right heel ; the toes of the two feet would be close together, left calf touching the right shinbone (tibia), knees well bent outward. (2) Without shifting the toes, dégagé on r.f. and raise left heel, thus rocking from l.f. to r.f. (3) Rock to the other foot. (4) Hop on l.f. and throw right leg to 2nd pos. elevation. The whole can now be reversed.

Berlin Polka.—Now obsolete. Position same as Pas de quatre. Consists of two parts. Bar 1 : Gentleman l.f., lady r.f. polka forward. Bar 2 : Counts 1, 2. Point inside foot to 4th position ; count 3, release hands, hop on other foot, turning half circle to face opposite direction. Bars 3. 4 : Repeat with opposite foot and moving in opposite direction and on the hop finish facing partner. Bars 5-8 : Polka. Repeat the whole *ad lib.*

Bocane (BO-KAHN).—This sedate dance for two persons in 2-4 tempo was first performed in 1646, and owes its name to Bocan, teacher of dancing to Anne of Austria, Charles I. of England, and most of the European Princesses Louis XIV. excelled in it as well as in the ballet " Cassandra," in which he made his debut at the age of 13. This young monarch excelled also in the ballet " de Flore," in the " Sissonne," " Bourrée," the gay " Rigodon d'Auvergne," the " Courante," the " Saraband " and Menuet. THE DANCE : For two people (1) both commence same foot. At first note of the music, glide r.f. forward, bending l. knee and inclining the body, raise yourself with the weight of the body on r.f.; this will give a salute forward. (2) glide l.f. forward as already explained, but in passing near the r. heel, the lady inclines her l. shoulder slightly towards the gentleman, the gentleman inclines his shoulder towards the lady ; this is the salute en passant (in passing) ; both draw upright, closing r.f. in front of l. Gentleman's r. hand takes partner's l. and she raises her skirt with the r. (3) commencing r.f. make three pas marchés forward, and pause with l.f. in rear for the 4th beat. (4) glide l.f. sideways and assemblé the heels. (5) glide l.f. forward, bending r. knee ; on the 3rd beat the r.f. closes up rear of l. heel. (6) take a step to rear with l.f. on beat 3, assemblé the heels. (7) glide r.f. forward, bending l. knee slightly; on the 3rd beat the l.f. closes up rear of r. heel. (8) repeat with r f. (9, 10, 11, 12) repeat 3, 4, 5, 6. (13) with r.f. repeat 7; release hands and lady raises skirt with both hands. (14) glide l.f. forward, slightly raising r.f. in rear ; on 3rd beat carry r.f. forward. (15) repeat the last. (16) assemblé, pause, and on 3rd beat, l.f. makes a step to rear, leaving r. toe on ground forward. (17) assemblé heels ; on 3rd beat glide l.f. forward. (18) four pas marchés, lady gives l. hand to gentleman. (19, 20. 21) repeat last three bars. (22) assemblé. (23 to 32) repeat twice from 13 to 17, the gentleman passes in front of the lady and both salute.

Boiteux (BWAH-TO). – Lame or limping ; this is therefore a hobbling step. From 1st position. (1) after a light hop on the l.f. extend r.f. forward. (2) put r.f. in 4th position forward. (3) dégagé, and carry l.f. forward a whole step. (4) put l.f. to 4th forward and dégagé. (5) hop on l.f. and prepare r.f. for next step. The step is always executed with the same foot. If done during a turn it is a *tour-boiteux.*

Another description : 1st position, after a very short *temps levé,* (1) glide r.f. to 4th position forward, dégagé. (2) l.f. to 1st position, first on the toes, but immediately by a sharp audible beat of the heel—*coup de talon*—in consequence of which the r.f. is liberated, leaves the ground, and, with a temps levé on the left, (3) and (4) follows with a pas glissé.

Bolero.—Derived from Volero owing to its grace and lightness. A noble Spanish dance for couples, vis-a-vis. Tempo 3-4. (Fig. 1) promenade. (Fig. 2) traversé ; lady and gentleman change places. (Fig. 3) avant deux. forward and return to places. (Fig. 4) la Finale, describe a circle. (Fig. 5) attitude.

Having executed some steps in place for 32 bars, they finish by assuming a noble attitude and agitating tambourines with both hands above the head, then strike the tambourines with the hands, the elbows, the knees, followed by port-de-bras, coupés, battements, lengthened glissades, terre-à-terre, glissé, frappés.

Bolero (another)— 120 bars in 3-4 tempo. By a couple vis-a-vis, holding tambourines in the r. hand raised above the head, left hand on the hips; in this way they walk in a circle, agitating the tambourines (8 bars). Both glide r.f. to right, draw l f. up to it, leaning head and body to left, shaking the tambourines (8 bars). Repeat with l.f , changing tambourines to other hands (8 bars). Change tambourines to r. hands. They join l. hands. Gentleman turns lady beneath l. arm *(allemande),* then release hands and the gentleman takes running steps round his partner, who still stands in attitude. He stops in front of her, and, giving the tambourine a tap with l. hand, assumes an attitude similar to hers (16 bars). Reverse the last movement, the lady dancing the gentleman's part and *vice versa* (16 bars). In this attitude they tap the tambourine for 32 bars, thus : they take it in l., and both tap with the r., the elbow, the hand, the head on l. side, the hand, the elbow, the hand, behind the back, one in front, on l. knee, on r. knee, then raising l. leg, passing both hands underneath, tap the tambourine, repeat with r. leg, lift the feet to the rear alternately and tap it with the heel, repeat with the toes forward, etc. They join r. hands, glide l.f. forward and stretch r.f. forward in the air, pass tambourine to other hand, joining l. hands; repeat with other hands; repeat three times with each foot—eight times altogether—and release hands. They run round each other, then retire to their original places and pivot there on one foot, while the other glides on the floor to the rear, making a circle. They move towards and face each other, execute a pas de valse from their places without turning, and starting with l.f. to left side, and transfering the weight of the body and arms to the left, and, shaking the tambourines, tap it with the left hand. Repeat with r.f.; with l.f.; the r. again. The lady now kneels on r. knee in attitude; the gentleman moves round her, tapping tambourine on various parts of his body. At the last note of the music he stands at rear of partner, in attitude, holding tambourine over head with both hands. They look at each other for the final salute on last note.

The Pas de Bolero employed for running or walking is the same as the backward or forward step of the Waltz and of the Boston. The tambourine must be shaken throughout the dance. The dance can be done by 1, 2, 4, 6 or 8 couples.

Bond (BON).—A springing movement. (*See* Bondir.)

Bondir (BON-DEER).—To bound, rebound or bounce. A great distinction must be drawn between springing (*bondir*) and jumping (*sauter*). In jumping, one remains in place; in springing, one leaves the spot from which the spring is made. *Un pas bondir* is therefore a springing *step*, causing the transfer of the weight of the body (dégagé). The spring refers to that foot which gives the impetus and is last on the floor. The free leg, which finally receives the weight of the body after the spring, either forward, backward or sideward, performs a *jété*. After the jèté, the other foot is free for the next step. "A child may be said to jump for joy, upon either or both feet, but in so doing remains on or near the place; while a man does not jump, but springs across a ditch; a sparrow jumps over a straw, a tiger springs at his prey." (*See* Jèté, Sauter.)

Boston.—The step of the Boston can best be defined as "two pas marchés and an assemblé." This is done forward, backward and in turning, at the dancer's will. The step *backward*: *First bar* (1) glide l.f. to 4th rear. (2) glide r.f. to 4th rear. (3) l.f. to 3rd forward. *Second bar* (1) glide r.f. to 4th rear. (2) glide l.f. to 4th rear. (3) r.f. to 3rd forward. The step *forward*: *First bar* (1) glide r.f. to 4th forward. (2) Glide l.f. to 4th forward. (3) r.f. to 3rd rear. *Second bar*, repeat, commencing left foot. To execute the step *in turning*, pivot a half-circle on the first beat of each bar. The music is the ordinary waltz, but the dance is done as though the music were written in 6-8 time. The ear must be closed to the rhythm of the waltz music, and the dance is executed to the rhythm of the dancer's personal taste and individuality. Having performed these steps a number of times the dancer introduces the following variation known as *The Run*. This is an ordinary walking step, thus: the gentleman Bostons backward (the lady forward) towards the centre—then a half-turn of Reverse Boston; the gentleman takes position at right side of lady, walk five steps forward (lady backward) and assemblé for the sixth beat and recommence the Boston step. Another variation which may be agreeably introduced is a sideward chassé. The variations are numerous, but the most important is the "DOUBLE BOSTON," as follows: *Gentleman's step* (1) strongly glide r.f. to rear. (2, 3) pivot a half-turn to left on the r.f.; during this turn the l.f. remains outstretched forward, toe down, and describes a half-circle at the same time as the body. (4) Glide l.f. strongly forward. (5) glide r.f. to the side. (6) Assemblé l.f. to r.f., again turning a half-circle to the left. *The Lady's step* is different. (1) glide l.f. forward. (2) glide r.f. to the right. (3) Assemblé l.f. to r.f., turning a half-circle. (4) glide r.f. backward. (5) glide l.f. (6) Assemblé r.f. to l.f., turning another half-circle. THE TRIPLE BOSTON—another variation—occupies four bars of music. *Gentleman's step*, first bar (1) glide l.f. forward (the gentleman being on the right of his partner, right shoulders almost touching). (2) glide r.f. forward. (3) glide l.f. forward. (The gentleman commences to alter his position to do the remaining steps on the left side of the lady). *Second bar* (1) glide r.f. forward (on the left side of the lady, l. shoulders almost touching). (2) glide r.f. forward. (3) Draw r.f. up to l.f.. *Third bar*, still on the l. side; (1) glide l.f. forward. (2, 3) pivot half-turn to left on the sole of l.f. *Fourth bar* (1) r.f. backward. (2,3) pivot a half-circle to left on the same foot; during this the gentleman places himself again on the r. side of the lady, to recommence the steps. The lady's step can be easily inferred from the gentleman's step; that is, she will make the steps (*pas marchés*) backward instead of forward, and then pivot twice like her partner.

Bouffons (danse des) (BOO-FON).—Tempus, Numa Papilius, second King of Rome, 714 to 671 B.C. Twelve men and women united to celebrate the sacred fête days of March. The Bouffons (jesters) danced to the sound of the bones.

Boulangère, *Baker* (BOO-LAHN-JHERE).—Ancient. All couples join hands in a circle, and move round, circling first to the right, then to the left. One couple then place themselves in centre. The gentleman turns his partner, who remains in the centre, and to whom he gives his r. hand. He turns the second lady with l. hand, returns to partner and turns with r.h.; then turns third lady with l. hand; and so on with all the ladies. When finished he returns with his partner to place. The circling round is repeated and another couple taking their places in the centre repeat the turns as before. This is repeated until all the couples have been in the centre.

Bourgeoise. (BOOR-JWAHZ).—XII Century. Tempo 3-4. Family dance in couples of the Bourgeoise (middle) class. They turned holding both hands, then clasping each other, glissés and chassés with each foot in turning.

Bourrée. (BOORAY).—A dance hailing from Auvergne and introduced to the French Court by Catherine de Medeci about 1565. Of a gay, rustic character.

Bourrée, pas de.—This means literally, a stuffing or crammed step and consists of three movements which adapt themselves in manifold forms to various dance-rhythms of ancient and modern times. Feuillet's "Choregraphie" mentions no less than ninety-three different Bourrées; this may be compared to a musical attempt to multiply the harmonies of three notes, upwards and downwards. It adapted itself to the gay rhythm of former fashionable dances, such as Anglaise, Allemande and Ecossaise, and as a rule with a preliminary *temps levé* was called in its time PAS FLEURET (probably because it resembled the steps employed in fencing). It was also called PAS COULÉ. The three steps of the Polka have been borrowed from this original pas, and even the chassé may be called a *syncopated pas de bourrée*. But, while there is a similarity between chassé and bourrée, there is in reality a marked difference. That which is "stuffed" or "crammed" (bourrée) is usually stationary, while that which is chased (chassé) is forced from its place: these characteristics apply to the two steps so named. In the forward bourrée, the free foot is brought against the supporting one which is held for a moment in position before it glides forward; in the forward chassé, the rear foot drives or chases the supporting foot from its place before receiving the weight. BOURRÉE EN AVANT :— Preparation—r.f. is put in 4th rear elevated position. With a light bend of the knee. (1) the r.f. is put into 4th forward position (a whole step). (2) l.f. to 3rd rear (a half step). (3) r.f. to 4th forward (a half step). BOURRÉE EN ARRIÈRE. Preparation—l.f. in 4th forward elevated position. The same three steps in a contrary movement, *i.e.* (1) l.f. to 4th rear. (2) r.f. to 3rd forward. (3) l.f. to 4th rear. When several pasi de bourrées follow each other forward and backward, the change of foot to the first of the three movements is absolutely necessary. BOURRÉE À CÔTÉ (sideward). Preparation— l.f. in 2nd point position. (1) l.f. to 3rd rear. (2) r.f. to 2nd. (3) l.f. to 3rd rear whilst r.f. is brought to 2nd point, ready to commence the following steps in the contrary direction. The movements should be executed on the floor and to one music tempo, by performing the 1st and 2nd steps in the first half beat, and the 3rd step in the full beat of the music; the accent is, therefore, on the 3rd step. The step may be done in turning, four pas bourrées en tournant should be sufficient for a complete tour (circle). BOURRÉE DESSOUS ET DESSUS (to rear and front). (1) the pointed l.f. falls to the rear (dessous) of the r.f. in 3rd position. (2) r.f. is placed in a very reduced position. (3) l.f. to 3rd front (dessus), r.f. assuming 2nd point position. It must be observed that all bourrées commence and end in open positions. BOURRÉE EN TRIOLE is the step executed in triole time; that is three triplets in a bar in 3-4 time, and the bourrée would then be made three times to a bar of music.

Bow.—The form of salutation by the gentleman equivalent to the lady's curtsey—technically, *révérence*. The custom of making a *révérence* each time a couple advances in square dances is superfluous. The salutation to partners and to centre at the beginning and end of a dance are sufficient. Repeated salutes during the figures are as superfluous as they would be in a social visit. Unfortunately, the ordinary bow, in the square dances, has degenerated into a vulgar nod or a tipping of the forefinger against the eye or some other part of the face. The bow properly executed should be—prepare by facing partner, and, while she curtseys to the left (*see* Curtsey), he bows to the left. (1) glide r.f. to 2nd, degagé. (2) glide l.f. to 3rd rear, simultaneously lowering the eyes, head and shoulders, body inclined forward and arms hanging loosely. (3, 4) slowly assume erect position. Bow to the right—(1) glide l.f. to 2nd, degagé. (2) glide r.f. to 3rd forward, and finish as before. (For explanation of bow to right and left *see* "Curtsey").

Bow-Legs and Knock-Knees (*Arqué et Jàrreté*).—Absolutely straight legs are very exceptional, few therefore can hold them straight with ease. Those whose knees nearly or quite touch, calves close together, while the heels are wide apart, are said to have narrow legs (*jàrreté*) or knock-knees. Such persons have large thick knees, and find great difficulty in standing with the heels together. *Bow-legged* (*arqué*) persons have a space between the knees, and the heels touch, these are called distant legs. Such people are peculiarly fitted for entrechats and similar steps in which the knees are often a hindrance in straight legs.

Brandons, Danse des.—XVI Century. This is still danced in various countries on the first Sunday in Lent. The peasants, with illuminated torches, dance round the bushes.

Branles (BRAHNL).—Period 996. Tempo 2-4. The Branles were very numerous, each having its distinguishing figure. It was danced singly and doubly. The most audacious of the Branles was "l'Antiquaille," which surpassed in boldness and immodesty the most daring Bourrée. The dancers in a circle, moved round singing. Then, releasing hands, they imitated, both in voice, movement and gesture, some animal or thing. One would pretend to be a galloping horse, another duelling, a drunken man or woman, etc.

Branle, pas de (double).—Glide l.f. to 2nd, draw r.f. to 3rd. Repeat. Repeat twice with the other foot. Repeat all. Raise and drop the r.f., then l.f., then r.f., followed by an attitude.

Branle de Poitou.—Under Charles IX, 1562. Common time. Three pas marchés and assemblé forward. Repeat to rear. Then each dancer imitates somebody or the capers of an animal according to choice.

Bras (BRAH).—THE ARMS. A gentleman should present his hand *supine* to the lady, that is, palm upward with the fingers slightly separated, the arm half extended and a slight inclination of the head. The lady presents her hand *prone*, that is, palm downward. The first four fingers of the lady are placed lightly on the gentleman's fingers, the thumbs lightly touching between the second and third fingers, gentleman's thumb on top and lady's underneath. He offers his r. arm half bent, raised level with the chest, which she accepts with the l., her arm being near his wrist.

Bras, Port de (PORT-DER-BRAH).—Carriage of the arms. Many systems have been employed in this branch of the Art, but that of the so-called French school has been most universally adopted. Certain alterations and additions to the French system are, however, necessary, and these changes are complimentary and not corrective. Such distinguished writers as Sulzer and Klemm have expressed themselves to that effect. The latter says, "Their systems might be employed, corrected and amplified by artistic masters, to assist in the advancement and development of the Art." Zorn says, "Our predecessors have achieved great results, and it is our duty to advance along the road which leads to the perfection of our art by means of the assistance they have left us; but it is a false admiration for that which has gone before which would prevent corrections or improvements; indeed, had all former writers clung to that line of action, we should still be dancing in the same manner as did Adam and Eve." The position, opposition and carriage of the arms are, perhaps, the three most difficult things in dancing, and, therefore, demand particular study and attention. Noverre, writing of opposition, says, "Of all the movements executed in dancing, the opposition or contrast of the arms to the feet is the most natural, and, at the same time, least attended to." The principle underlying "opposition" is a law of equilibrium. In walking, when the r.f. is forward the l. arm is also forward, when the l.f. is forward the r. arm is forward.

The old FRENCH SYSTEM of Arm positions.—1st position, arms hanging normally perpendicularly at the side. 2nd position, arms held out horizontally at the side. 3rd position, arms held out in front, fingers almost touching. 4th position, arms held out straight horizontally in front. 5th position, arms perpendicularly over the head, tips of fingers touching.

The system advocated by Zorn has much to recommend it. He describes a circle, having the neck as the centre and the finger tips the circumference. Raising the arms from the perpendicular hanging to the perpendicular overhead, one would describe this circle, which he divides as follows:—Arms hanging are in 1st *position*; level with shoulders are in *3rd position*; straight overhead are in *5th position*; midway between 1st and 3rd will be *2nd*; midway between 3rd and 5th will be *4th*. Mathematically, this is correct and is a commonsense view. The arms then could be in these positions: side, front or rear; example—*Arms 3rd position side* would be, the arms held out horizontally to the side, level with the shoulders; *arms 3rd position front*, the arms held out horizontally in front; *intermediate 3rd*, between side and front; *arms 4th position side*, they would be held up aloft obliquely sideways between the horizontal and perpendicular; *4th position front* would bring them obliquely forward, etc. One arm could then be in one position, while the other arm is in another position. Thus, l. arm could be 4th side and r. arm 3rd front. It must, however, be remembered that the fully stretched arm is seldom employed in dancing. There are, therefore, five degrees of bending the arm—(a) *tendu*, fully stretched; (b) *demi-tendu*, half-stretched, *i.e.* arm slightly bent; (c) *arrondi*, rounded (the most generally used); (d) *demi-courbé*, half-bent; (e) *courbé*, quite bent. The fingers should always hang loosely. The arm placed with hand hanging over the head (as in Scotch dances) would be *side 4th arrondi*; the other hand on the hip would be *side 2nd demi-courbé*. Example—assuming the position desired is r. arm in front of the body, level with chest, and hand hanging, this would be *3rd front position courbé*. Resumé—1st *arm position*, arms at the side, hanging naturally. *2nd arm position*, arms, though hanging, form an oval with elbows well-turned out. *3rd arm position*, arms raised to height of shoulder held out in an open circle. *4th arm position*, arms held rounded with hands hanging so that the tips of the fingers will be above the ears. *5th arm position*, arms are raised, rounded, over the head, the tips of the middle fingers nearly touching. Positions may be found in which the arm is bent and the hand resting on the hip, this is called *demi-bras*.

Brisé (BREEZAY).—Literally, broken. A temps and a pas. Somewhat similar to entrechat, but in the latter, both feet are in action; in brisé, one foot is in action, the other merely helps. During a hop on one foot, the other foot beats dessus and dessous or dessous and dessus then receiving the weight of the body. If there is no transfer of weight (*degagé*) it is a *temps brisé*. If, after the transfer, the movement is repeated with the other foot, it is *brisé alternatif*. A brisé can be concluded on either or both feet. The movement is a rapid zig-zag cut as distinct from a coupé, which is a straight cut.

27

BR

PRONOUNCING DICTIONARY OF

Brisé moucheté (MOOSHERTAY).— *Blunted.* With r.f. in 4th forward, make an echappé, and, with a slight hop on r.f., raise l.f. in a battement plié backward, then with another slight hop on r.f., the l.f. makes another battement plié forward, then a jeté in the rear raising the r., and finish with assemblé. This step can also be done turning. BRISÉ BATTU. - With l.f. in 5th rear, bend slightly, raise the heel, and making a hop, beats stretched above r.f. and falls to the ground with the weight, and the r.f. is in 5th forward. From this position the pas can be repeated, gaining ground. The feet must fall to the ground one after the other; should they fall simultaneously it will not be a brisé. BRISÉ VOLÉ.—(*Flying*). The same as the foregoing, but in this, the second foot in not placed on the ground. With r.f. raised in rear, hop and beat the foot in front of l.f. and fall with weight on r.f., raising l.f. crosswise forward in the air—this is brisé volé forward. To execute it to the rear, throw l.f. rapidly to the rear, the remainder of the step as before. BRISÉ SIGNÉ.—Raising l.f. from 5th rear, stretch it suddenly, and, during a hop on r.f., throw it to 2nd position, the r.f. falling immediately in 5th forward. (This will make the sign of the brisé instead of beating it). The movement can be repeated. BRISÉ VOLÉ MARQUÉ. —(*Marked*). The body turns in the direction in which the pas is taken; with l.f. raised in rear, make a jeté to 2nd position, raising r.f. to 4th forward. Throw r.f. with a jeté to rear, raise l.f. to 4th rear, throw it again forward and r.f. in rear, thus making them volés instead of battus.

Brydalica.—Ancient Greek dance by men masked as grotesque women. It was wanton and indecent.

Buffalo.—A dance of the Red Indians. Represents a grand hunt. One of the braves fixes the skull and horns of a buffalo on his head and skips about as the others try to catch him, dancing the while.

Byllichal.—Ancient Greek dance quoted, without any comment, by Pollox.

C

Cabaratière.—A dance of the Middle Ages. It sometimes substituted the first steps of the Menuet as danced at the Middle-class balls. None of the theory is in existence, only the name remains.

Cabriole (KAH-BREE-OLE) or Capriole.—A term borrowed by the French, from the Italian "capriola." The crossing of both feet, which was adopted about 1730 by the renowned dancer Camargo, was called *capriola intrecciata*, interwoven caprioles, and from this originate the terms "cabriole" and "entrechat." In the old Italian School (which the French adopted) the springing of both legs in the air, combined with battements in the air, was called "capriola," and the French in adopting it employ the technical term "*friser la cabriole*," "curl the cabriole." It was also called "quinte." Costa's "Treatise on the Art of Dancing" (Turin, 1831) says, "It will be well to give a rule as to the manner of counting the cuts in the interwoven caprioles, called by the French *entrechat*. In whichever manner these Entrechats are executed, the closed and open cuts are counted together and one must pass through the second position to make a battement in the fifth. Standing with l.f. in forward 5th position. (Cut 1) leap with both feet; (cut 2) the l. strikes the r. below, the r. simultaneously strikes the l. above; (cut 3) reopen the feet in 2nd position; (cut 4) fall with l.f. in 5th forward position: all

28

this during one spring. Thus, during a single spring in the air, strike or twirl the legs and feet together, crossing and recrossing them as often as possible, making as many entrechats as can be made in one jump. The crossings of the legs are termed "*trioles*," and are performed during the jump, finishing in either an open or closed position. Sometimes, springing from the floor, striking the two heels together and alighting on one foot is called a cabriole. (*See* Entrechat.)

Cachucha or **Catchucha** (KA-CHEW-KA).—A Spanish (Andalusian) national solo dance for a lady, with castagnets. Cachucha means anything pretty or an attractive bauble. The dance is one of grace, gaiety and passion. The music, in 3-8 tempo, consists of two parts of eight bars each, which are played four times and coda. The play of the castagnets, the movements of the body and arms in opposition, the pleasant facial expression, the whole producing a vivid picture of grace and elegance, are essential features of the dance.

THE DANCE.— Prelude, chords, FIRST COUPLET, four figures of 16 bars each.

Figure 1. Zig-zag forward (*ballonné progressif*, 16 bars). Enter from rear diagonally forward to right with *three ballonnés dessous, one pirouette* and *one frappé dessus* into 5th position (4 bars). Repeat to left (4 bars). Repeat to right (4 bars). Repeat left to centre (4 bars).

Figure 2. Pivoter, 16 bars. Turn slowly backward to left in place with *six pas de ciseaux dessous* in 2nd and 5th positions, with l. arm raised (6 bars). *Pas de basque pirouette* to left (2 bars). Repeat to right (8 bars).

Figure 3. Zig-zag backward with *ballonné retrograde* (16 bars). One *ballonné* to right followed raising into 5th point and audible lowering of r. heel, and carry l.f. into 2nd elevation (1 bar). Put down l.f. in 2nd position. Glide r. into 5th front, pointing toe strongly down, audibly lowering the heel, immediately carrying l.f. into rear elevation. Carry l.f. to 2nd, dégagé (1 bar). During this bar the r. arm executes a large arm-circle (*grand rond de bras*), accompanied by such a bend of the body that the r. hand nearly touches the floor, and then a corresponding movement of the l. arm. Carry r.f. to 2nd dégagé. Execute a complete turn (*tour entier*) on r. ball, carrying l.f. first into 2nd elevation and then into 5th front position and dégagé (1 bar). Round sole of r.f. into front 5th dégagé. Pause (1 bar). Begin *ballonné* as preparation for the repetition (1 bar). Repeat this *ballonné retrograde* (4 bars) to left. Repeat the whole enchaînement (8 bars).

Figure 4. *Frappé tortillé* in the background, 16 bars. *Traversé* to right sideways with one *frappé* and one *tortillé*, repeated three times, followed by one *coupé* and one *pas de basque latéral.* (1) *frappé* with r.f. into 2nd dégagé. (2) turn l.f. on the heel until the toe comes to a point a little in advance of the r. heel. (3) turn l.f. into front 5th position. (2 *and* 3 *constitute a pas tortillé*) (1 bar). Repeat twice (2 bars). (1) *coupé dessous* with r.f. into 5th rear. (2) l.f. to 2nd dégagé. (3) r.f. to front crossed 4th position, dégagé (1 bar) (*this constitutes a pas de basque espagnol*) Repeat the preceding 4 bars to left (4 bars). Repeat them to right (4 bars). *Two frappés tortillés* (2 bars). *Coupé pas de basque* (1 bar). (1)

frappé on r.f. into front 4th dégagé. (2) pause. (3) prepare for next movement (1 bar).

SECOND COUPLET. Four figures of 16 bars each.

Figure 1. *Le rhombe en descendant,* (16 bars). Obliquely forward to right to the middle line by one and a half *ballonnés,* two *pas éléves* forward into 4th position, one *demi-pas-de-basque* to the left, one *tappé du talon gauche* (stamp with l. heel) and one *frappé* with r.f. into 2nd position (4 bars). It would be to the advantage of the pupil to divide the counting of the next four bars, from 1 to 12. (1) After a light hop on l.f. put down r.f. in 2nd dégagé, r. hand over the head, eyes raised to upstretched hand. (2) l.f. to 3rd rear. (1, 2 *constitute a pas ballonné*). (3, 4) repeat 1, 2. (5, 6) two *pas éléves* on line of direction. (7) l.f. to 2nd. (8) swing r f. into crossed front 4th position. (7, 8 *constitute a demi-, or half-pas-de-basque.* and many Spanish dancers call it *pointe de pied*). (9) Raise l. heel and audibly lower it, this is known as stamping, or *taper.* (10) stamp with r.f. into 2nd dégagé. (11, 12) pause (4 bars). Repeat 1 to 12 with opposite feet, obliquely forward. Repeat with r.f. obliquely backward ; in doing this the dancer turns her back to the audience (4 bars). Repeat once more (4 bars), finish facing audience.

Figure 2. Sixteen *demi-pas-de-basques* with *tapés de talon,* bringing the dancer to front of stage (16 bars).

Figure 3. *Le rhombe en montant.* The same as Figure 1 of this couplet, except that it is backward (16 bars).

Figure 4. In the foreground. *Demi-traversé a droit,* consisting of *coupé-tortillé, coupé-pas-de-basque, frappé-ramassé* and *frappé-pirouette.* (1) *coupé :* put l.f. down forcibly in rear 5th dégagé. (2) *tortillé :* turn r.f. inward on the ball. (3) turn r.f. outward into front 5th dégagé. (4) *coupé :* put down l.f. forcibly into 5th rear and dégagé, thus releasing r.f. (5) *pas de basque :* carry r.f. to 2nd position and dégagé. (6) carry l.f. by a circular movement into 4th front position, dégagé. (7) *frappé :* stamp with r.f. into 2nd position, dégagé. (8) *ramassé :* bend supporting r. leg and glide l f. into front 5th point with corresponding bend of l. leg, simultaneously bend body, dipping l. arm, so that it would be possible for the l. hand to lift a small object from the floor ; "*ramasser*" means to pick up. The r. arm during this movement is raised to a corresponding position in the opposite direction ; the eyes follow the movement of the l. hand. (9) put down the l. and raise r. heel, straighten the body, commencing a dégagé, which is completed on (10) by a stamp with r.f. in 2nd position. (11) raise r. heel and execute a complete turn to the r. upon the sole, with l. leg in 2nd elevation. (12) put down l.f. in 2nd position, dégagé (4 bars in all). *Retraversé :* repeat the same enchaînement but in counter-motion (4 bars). Repeat to right (4 bars). Repeat to left to centre but without *ramassé* (4 bars).

THIRD COUPLET. Four figures of 16 bars each.

Figure 1. *Ballonné retrograde* zig-zag backward ; same as 3rd figure of 1st couplet. (16 bars).

Figure 2. In the background in place. Three *temps de ciseaux,* without hop or turn, one *coupé* and one *pas de basque* to the right (4 bars). Repeat (4 bars). *Pivoter* to left, with l. arm raised and *pirouette basque* to left, as in 2nd figure of 1st couplet (8 bars).

Figure 3. Zig-zag forward with two successive *pirouettes* After a light hop (1–4) move obliquely forward to the right, halfway to centre, by one-and-a-half *pas ballonnés*. (5) complete turn on r. ball, with l.f. in 5th rear elevation with perpendicular sole. (6) put down l.f. in front 5th. (7) stamp r. in 2nd position, dégagé. (8, 9, 10) repeat 5, 6, 7. (11, 12) pause. (The whole, 4 bars). Repeat this enchaînement to left (4 bars). Repeat the whole (8 bars).

Figure 4. *Ramassé* (16 bars). Short zig-zag to rear with eight raising and picking-up movements, in six beats. Preparation : *temps levé* (this consists of a *fouetté* and a hop preparatory to the *pas ballonné*). (1) put down r.f. in 2nd position. (2) *ramassé* (already explained). (3) put down l.f. and raise r. heel. (4) stamp with r.f. into 2nd position: (5) *temps fouetté dessous*, whipping leg in rear. (6) *temps levé*, as used to prepare for a *pas ballonné*. This enchaînement of six temps is repeated alternately eight times (16 bars in all), and brings the dancer to the centre of the background.

FOURTH COUPLET.

Figure 1. *Grand dégagé*, zig-zag forward. (1–4) move obliquely forward to right, halfway to centre, with one-and-a-half *pas ballonnés*. (5–6) one-and-a-quarter turns on r. sole with l.f. in high 2nd elevation. (7) l.f. down to 4th front position, raising l. arm and following its movement with the eyes. (8) dégagé slowly and with dignity to l.f., same time bend upper body, lowering l. arm and raising r. arm and bending the knees. (9) repeat with r.l. (10) repeat 7. (11, 12) pause. (The whole four bars). Music from 5 to 12 should be *rallentando*. All the movements should be executed in an easy, airy manner, with corresponding arm movements. Repeat to left forward (4 bars). Repeat to left forward (4 bars). Repeat to right forward (4 bars). Repeat to left forward, kneeling slowly on l. knee during the 16th bar, with r. arm lowered and l. arm raised, head slightly inclined forward, eyes downcast.

Figure 2. *Dégagé à genoux.* (Transfer upon the knees, 16 bars). During first four bars, carry r. arm inside the r. leg by a *grand rond de bras*, which then moves upward, and through a raised position returning again lowered outside the r. leg, accompanied by a similar but opposite movement with l. arm. The eyes follow r. hand, head and body inevitably coöperate (4 bars). During the 5th bar, carry l. arm to crossed horizontal position, turn upper body slightly to left, eyes following l. hand, rise slowly on r.f. during bar 6, continuing the movements of the arms. During 7th bar carry r.f. to 2nd dégagé, and with l.f. make a *jeté en tournant*, sinking, during the 8th bar, on the r. knee. Repeat the whole, opposite way (7 bars), rising on 8th bar.

Figure 3. In the foreground. One-and-a-half *pas ballonnés* and two *pas éléves* to the right (2 bars). Deep curtsey to audience on right (2 bars). Repetition to left (4 bars). Backward to centre with two-and-a-half *pas ballonnés* in circular direction to right, and a complete turn to right on right sole, and low curtsey to centre of audience. (8 bars).

Coda. The dancer concludes with one-and-a-half *pas ballonnés* and several *pas éléves* to left and exit on last note of music.

Cadence.—From *cadere*, to fall. The observance of the minutest rhythm of the pas with the rhythm of the music. It denotes the harmony of the dancer with the accompanying music. Commonly known as "keeping time."

Cagneux (KAHN-YO).—Knock-kneed. A dancer whose knees turn inward, that is, they nearly touch each other. This fault is fatal to the training of a good dancer, because there appears to the onlooker, a disagreeable contraction of the thighs and hips, and, instead of the legs being straight, they form a triangle, with the knees as the apex and the feet for the base. The remedy, which must be steadily persevered with, is an extended course of *grands ronds de jambe* (rounding the leg in the air). The practice of these ronds produces equality of the rotary movement of the femir bone in the cup-shaped cotyloid cavity. The patella (knee-pan) will then move to the side, and will, little by little, become perpendicular with the toes.

Caledonians.—Once a popular Square Dance, now almost obsolete. Arrangement of dancers as for Quadrilles.

Figure 1. First and second couples advance to the centre and *demi-moulinet* (half-mill) to left (join r. hands across and walk round to left). Change hands and *demi-moulinet* to right, and back to places. *Balancez* (set to) and turn partners : ladies chain. Half promenade. *Demi-* (half) *chaine Anglaise* (half right and left). Sides repeat.

Figure 2. First gentleman advance and retire twice, All *balancez* and turn corners, gentleman keeping corner lady. All promenade once round. Repeat—second gentleman commencing. Repeat for third gentleman, and again for the fourth.

Figure 3. Same as 1st Figure of Lancers, and add Grand Circle and turn partners.

Figure 4. First lady and *vis-a-vis* (opposite gentleman) advance to centre and stop. Partners repeat. Turn partners to places. All ladies walk round four steps into the places of the ladies on the right. All salute. Gentlemen walk round four steps into places of gentlemen on the left. All salute. Repeat the last two movements. Promenade to place. Repeat the whole, the second lady and her *vis-a-vis* commencing. Repeat, third lady commencing, and again for fourth lady.

Figure 5. First couple promenade 16 steps round the set. All ladies advance and retire (en avant et en arrière) bowing. All gentlemen advance to the centre and face partners, salute. *Balancez* to (set) partners and turn. Half grand chain. Promenade to places. *Chassez croisés* with corners. Repeat the whole three times for the second, third and fourth couples to commence in turn.

Calife, le (KAH-LEEF).—An ancient contredanse composed by Blasis for four couples. (1) a gentleman advances and retires alone. (2) the *vis-a-vis* lady repeats. (3) the same for the other three ladies together, who make a chassé croisé, finishing vis-a-vis to the gentleman. (4) the gentleman advances with the three ladies, makes a *tour de main* (circle round holding hands) and all return to places. (5) the gentleman makes a balancé and *tour de main* with his partner and chassé sideward. Repeat.

Callichoré.—The name of a well, and of a dance. The ancient Greek womens' dance round the well of that name. Singing accompanied the dance.

Cambré, *pas* (KAHM-BRAY).—With military salute. Open the heels and pivot on the toes; the points are inward, the feet in the form of an arch, toes nearly touching in front, heels open in the rear. Raise the shoulders while making a military salute. Then pivot on the heels, opening the toes (the feet thus assuming the 2nd position) and assemblé, letting the hands fall.

Canaica.—Russian. The couples surrender themselves to graceful balancés; it is a kind of valse with change of hands, intermingled with forward and backward promenades.

Canaries.—XVI Century. Tempo 6-8. A species of Jig for two people, danced in the Canary Islands (*authority*, Compan). It was drawn from a ballet or masquerade, in which the dancers were dressed as Kings of Mauritius or savages with feathers of all colours. It was lively and animated. Thoinot-Arbeau, in his "Orchéso-graphie" (1588), gives this explanation of the dance. "A young man takes a girl, and they dance to the rhythm of any tune they like. He conducts her to the end of the ballroom and either withdraws or recommences. They dance again and he again withdraws, then she dances alone before him and retires to her place. They continue in this way as long as the music suggests anything, some of the passages being strange, eccentric, and almost savage."

Another description.—The dancers place themselves opposite to each other, imitating savages. The man places his arm round the woman and they dance together a *pas de gigue burlesque.* They separate and execute a *pas de navette* (going and returning), imita-ting a person wiping his shoes on the floor. Then they recommence, the woman halts at a corner of the room, and her partner, with a savage mien, executes a solo while pretending to search for her. Then he repeats the tapping etc., commencing with the other foot. Then commence from the beginning, and this time the woman does the solo, etc.

Canaries, pas de.—Tap with l.f., lifting the r., tap with r. heel, then stamp with whole foot. Repeat.

Cancan or Chahut.—A kind of frenzied, epileptic or mad dance. The movements are about as related to dancing as slang is to refined language. The Cancan does not form a part of any musical law, but is the result of the temperament of the dancers, in their frantic efforts to give exhibitions of agility and suppleness. It is doubtful whether the Cancan of 1505 has any connection with the modern Cancan, which dates from 1830, when dancing in France was indulged in only by the lower classes. The process of transforma-tion by the lower orders continued until 1840. At first, the dance was far from coarse or licentious; it was graceful, even spiritual. By 1844, it was danced only by the young students at their evening frivolities at places like Mabille, Prado and Chaumière. Few of the better class indulged in the coarseness of this famous quadrille. The monstrous contortions of the votaries of the dance at Moulin Rouge are indescribable, they are anything but the joyful expres-sions of youth. The most horrible contortions and daring gestures were seen, and it is not surprising that the young students soon became satiated and wearied of this dance. Various unsuccessful attempts have been made to revive the Chahut or Cancan, but the condemnation of its monstrosities by the Press, and the articles and drawings by Louis Legrand in "Gil Blas" during May, 1891, finally effected the suppression of this horrible dance. It never had a strong footing in England, and, in its day, was seen here only on the music hall stage, never in the ballroom.

Candiote.—Greek dance (1623), based on a tender and languorous air. A young girl conducts various figures by circuits, voltes, ronds, etc., the dancers following the détours of a labyrinth, in a word, to represent the episode of Thesée and Ariadne. Homer wrote this description:—" Young men and girls, joining hands, dance together. The girls are clothed in light materials, on their heads are golden crowns. The young men are arrayed in brilliant colours. A troupe of these dance round in a circle of perfect precision, a perfect wheel. The circle opens, and the leading girl conducts the young people, who are still holding hands, through an infinite variety of turns." The dance was used by the Greeks at their rustic fêtes (fêtes champêtres). Compare with the later " Farandole," and note the similarity.

Cantique.—Dance, with song, used by the Ancient Hebrews. The Israelites, during the passage of the Red Sea, danced clasping one another, jumping and singing. It was the dance in the history of Palestine, 2,300 years B.C.

Caprice (KAH-PREES).--1821. Dance in imitation of the capricious goat, dancing and leaping. Eight bars, common time. The gentleman clasping the lady, they make four glides with each foot (4 bars), then four turns of a kind of hop waltz, jumping (4 bars), then they unclasp and do the movements separately, then together again, etc.

Carmagnole (la) (KARMAHNYOL).—Dates from August, 1789, in France. Carmagnole is an Italian town which was occupied by the French in 1581, 1671 and 1796. The French caused the inhabitants of Carmagnole to dance, and, chasing them out, occupied their town. Hence the name Carmagnole, which has been given to the steps of this dance, inspired the conqueror with joy and the vanquished with sorrow, despair and the desire for vengeance. Hence the saying when a man wants to fight another, " Je vais te faire danser la Carmagnole," (" I am going to make you dance the Carmagnole.") It was danced in the public places after the taking of the Bastille, July 14th, 1789, when it was made into a round dance, all singing the song, " La Carmagnole."

The Dance. One turn with the r. arms locked, hopping on l.f., and crossing r.f. in front of it; repeat three times. One turn with l. arms locked. One turn, holding both hands. The man with woman's l. hand in his r., taps one foot on the ground, and, raises the other; repeat three times. Then, facing each other, they give both hands and repeat the steps with the opposite feet. Then all joined hands in a huge circle, and performed a mad galop about the streets in a kind of Farandole. The circles were formed round the dwellings of the aristocrats to give expression of their horror at the inmates. The Jacobins excelled at it in the taking of the Bastille. Woe betide the aristocrat whose residence was so surrounded, he and his family were doomed !

Carré (KAR-RAY).—A square. The form in which square dances are arranged.

Carriage.—Correct carriage of the body is of the utmost importance to the dancer. The head must be held erect, eyes directed straight forward, neck perpendicular, chest expanded and forward, shoulders held back and down, arms hanging at the side with fingers rounded, abdomen drawn in, knees turned outward and stretched, legs and feet turned outwards.

Caryates.—Dance of ancient Greece. Combines great nobility and virginal innocence. It was reserved for the virgins of Lacome, who were proud in having acquired it from Pollux himself. The young maidens danced the caryates with the Spartans round the altar of Diana. Helène was the principal ornament of the fête, and it is said that it was at a caryates that the son of Priam became enamoured of her.

Cascaron.—" Le Figaro," of March, 1891, ascribes this dance to Mexico, where it was invented in honour of the Spanish-American Colony The lady chose a partner by drawing, from a satin satchel, a gilded and perfumed paper, which she threw over his head. There is a modern figure ("the snow-ball") in the Cotillon, which is identical with it. The lady, placed in the centre of the ballroom. surrounded by a group of gentlemen, breaks a ball containing confetti over him whom she desires as a partner.

Casse-Cou (*pas du*) (KAHS-KOO).—Break neck or dare-devil. Lower the head forward, raising the feet one after the other to the rear; then lifting the feet forward one after the other and hopping.

Cat's-Tail.—See *Chat, queue de.*

Centre of Gravity.—The proper balance of the body is the *sine qua non* of the dancer both on the stage and in the ballroom. The dancer must have absolute control of the movements of his own body before he is capable of properly guiding or sustaining a partner. The centre of gravity is at the base of the vertebral column. Whatever the position of the body, whatever movement the body may make, whether on one leg or both, the centre of gravity must never be altered. The weight of a dancer on one leg is divided in two equal parts to the weight which supports the whole. In this position, the line of the centre of gravity passes the axis of the leg which supports the body. Theatrical dancers must take into account the slope of the stage which descends in an inclined plane towards the spectators, which causes the body to incline forward. To counteract this, the head must be held high, and the body well back, so that the crown of the head is perpendicular with the slope of the loins.

Chacone (SHAH-KON).—Tempo 2-4. Has been danced since 1750. It was a dance indefinitely prolonged. Its name, originally Ciaccono, was derived from Ciécos, a blind man. It was first danced at the beginning of XVII. century. It originated in Italy at the time of the marriage of Marie de Medecis with Henry IV. in 1600, but according to Cervantes, Ménage, and others, the Chacone is really Spanish. According to Cervantes the Chacone was primitively danced by the negroes and mulattos, and imported by them to the Court of Philip II, but Castilian gravity singularly modified its character. It is admittedly a noble dance, and such musicians as Lulli, Berton, Rameau and Floquet did not disdain to write exquisite music for it. *Analysis:*—L.f. forward 5th, with weight of body on it. L.f. assemblé after r.f. has been raised to 2nd elevation, then bend (*plier*), draw upright with a hop on l.f. (*sauté*). The r. leg, which was *en l'air* (in the air), is carried to one side in 2nd position, and l.f. is placed either front or rear, according to the direction to be taken. This is the step in the Chaconne employed for the dancer to move either to the right or left.

Chaconne (*temps de*).—The name given to the whole of the above movements. The Chaconne easily adapts itself to either 2-4 or 3-4 tempo. Summary :—*Sauté* and two *pas marchés* on the points, which can be *rallentando* (slower) or *accellerando* (quicker) according to the music tempo.

Chaîne (SHAYN).—A figure in which the hands are alternately given in meeting another dancer. Of these figures there are several: *chaîne anglaise* (commonly known as "right and left") ; *chaîne des dames* (ladies chain) ; *chaîne en trois, en quatre, en six, en huit* (chain for three, four, six or eight) ; *grande chaîne* (grand chain); *chaîne en ligne* (chain in line). When a number of couples walk round in an inverse sense, as in 5th figure of Lancers (gentleman moving round the circle to the right and ladies to the left) and presenting alternately the l. hand and r. hand to each dancer, in passing round either to left or right of the other dancer, it is called *grande chaîne*. Two ladies meet in the centre of the set, taking r. hands and pass on with l. hand to opposite gentleman and return to places in the same way will be *chaîne des dames* (ladies' chain). It is a double when done by four people, when it is also called *moulinet* (moolinay) *a mill*. A complete *chaîne* occupies eight bars of music, and finds the dancers in their places ; a *demi-chaîne*, or half chain, takes four bars, and leaves the dancer into the opposite place.

Chaîne Anglaise (SHAYN AHNGLAYZ).—English chain. The familiar right and left in figures of square dances. (*See* Quadrilles).

Chaîne Brisé (SHAYN BREEZAY). In the grand chain, when gentleman meets his partner on the opposite side, he often executes a turn holding r. hands.

Chaîne Continué.—By two couples. The two ladies join r. hands and place l. hands in partner's hands, releasing the r. The gentlemen join r. hands and take the l. hands of opposite lady. Repeat the whole to return to place.

Chaîne des dames (SHAYN DAY DAHM).—Ladies chain. (*See* Quadrilles).

Champêtre (SHARMPAYTR).—Rural or country dances. Annually performed in the country. These dances are of great antiquity, but have now completely altered their character, in fact, have lost their originality. In former times the youth, and often the adults, fêted the village saint by dancing and rejoicing in the open air. The coming of spring, harvesting and other operations, gave opportunity for such rejoicing by the populace, in the open, under the light of the moon and stars, free to everybody. Now, one pays for admission into some theatre to see a few children gamboling in a supposed revival of dances, which were never intended to be danced on boards, but in the fields. They were instituted by the god Pan, who desired them to be danced in the woods. The dancers were garlanded with flowers, and wore sashes of blossoms.

Changement (SHAHNJ-MAHN).—Change. In marching or walking, when one is " out of step," and a change of step is necessary (1) step forward on r. or l. (and) close other foot up to it in 3rd position. (2) step forward again with first foot.

Changement de Jambe (SHAHNJ-MAHN DER JHAHMB).—Change of leg. The crossed changing of both feet in the air in one temps. With r.f. in 5th front, after a slight bend of the knees, give a moderate spring in the air and change the feet to l.f. in 5th front. It can also be done in turning.

Changement de Pieds (PER-AY).—Change of feet. Same as the foregoing.

Changement de Talons (TAH-LORN).—Change of heels. In right front 3rd position ; rise on the points and pass l. heel in front of r.f. and r. heel behind l.f. (ensemble). This may be repeated.

Changement le Main.- Change from one hand to the other.

Chao (KAH-O).—Very popular Chinese dance, done by a man playing an instrument resembling the figure 2, hence the origin of the name

Charisia (KAH-RIS-YER).—A fête, instituted, as its name indicates, in honour of the graces. Young men and maidens danced, offering each other cakes and fruits. It was always danced after sunset.

Charmeuse (LA) —(A New Ballroom dance by Bernard Leefson of Amsterdam). This dance consists of three parts of 16 bars each in Mazurka time. The lady and gentleman stand side by side in the 3rd position, the l.f. in front. The lady's l. hand in the gentleman's r. Both hands are raised to the height of the shoulder, the arm is gracefully bent. The gentleman places the l. hand akimbo, the lady holds her skirt with her r. hand, and before beginning the dance, both curtsey.

No. 1. Four Pas de Basque forward, beginning with the l.f. (4 bars). The gentleman makes his lady perform a *Tour de Valse* inward and outward, without unclasping his hand (4 bars). The gentleman is now standing in the 2nd position the weight of the body on the l. leg, the lady passes under the gentleman's arm. Both Waltz round, the gentleman beginning with l.f., the lady with the r.f. (8 bars).

No. 2. Placed as in No. 1. The gentleman begins with the l.f., the lady with the r., both make *Two Balancés* sideward (2 bars). In executing the first *Balancé*, they turn a little away from each other ; in making the 2nd, they incline a little towards each other, and describe an elegant curve with the arm. Make a *Tour de Valse* turning round each outside and release the hands (2 bars). *Waltz* as No. 1 (4 bars). Repetition of the same part (8 bars).

No. 3. The lady places herself opposite the gentleman, who stands with the back turned to the middle of the room. The gentleman offers his right hand to the lady who places hers in his Perform *Balancé* forward and backward, both beginning with the r.f. Position as in menuet (2 bars). Half *tour de main* (Waltz) (2 bars). Repetition of the Balancé, the l. hands being clasped together (2 bars). Half *tour de main* (Waltz) to the left (2 bars). The gentleman beginning with the l.f. *Waltz* as in No. 1.

The numbers follow in this order :

No. 1. Once.	*No. 1. Once.
No. 2. Twice.	No. 3. Twice.

*Before the repetition of No. 1, the lady and gentleman make two steps. (Marché à la Menuet) 2 bars, the gentleman beginning with the l.f., the lady with the r. one, and curtsey to each other.

Chassé, *pas* (SHAHS-SAY).—The chasing of one foot from its place by the other foot in two steps—one complete step and two half-cut steps—in two temps. It can be executed in all directions, forward, backward, to right, to left, and turning. *Analysis:—En avant* (forward); feet in forth position, weight on l.f. (1) r.f. to 4th forward, dégagé, and after a light bending and rising, is chased from its position by the l.f., which assumes the 3rd position rear of the r.f., while (2) the r.f. glides lightly forward to 4th position. This can be continued or *chassé alternatif*, by alternatively chasing the r.f. and l.f. *En arrière*; chase the foot backward. It can be done in either 2-4 or 3-4. Old-time contre-danses were executed with chassés combined with glissades, jetés, and assemblés.

Chassé Battu (SHAHS-SAY BAHTTU).—Beaten chassé. With r.f. in 5th forward, make an *echappé* on l.f. while r.f. makes a *battement plié* forward; while making a *jeté* forward with r.f. the l.f. makes a *battement plié* to rear, returning to 4th rear.

Chassé et Déchassé.—Chassé'to right and left, or *vice versa*.

Chassé Croisé.—In making the chassé to the right, the gentleman passes behind the lady, who simultaneously chassez to the left, passing in front of the gentleman, and, in returning to places, the gentleman chassez to left behind the lady, who does it to right, in front of the gentleman. It usually occupies eight bars of music.

Chassé Échappé (AY-SHAHP-AY) —With r.f. in 5th forward (1) make an échappé. (2) l.f. goes to 5th rear. (3) r.f. goes to 2nd. (4) quickly place l.f. in 5th forward.

Chassé Ouvert (OO-VAIR).—Two bars in 3-4 or 6-8 time. To the right. Glide r.f. forward, chasser r.f. with the l f., crossing it to the rear to glide l.f. to 2nd position. Chasser l.f. with r.f. in crossing r.f. behind l.f. and assemblé l.f. behind r.f. For CHASSÉ-OUVERT-BATTU make an assemblé, preceded by an entrechat or brisé. This step is repeated, commencing l.f. (2 bars).

Chat, *pas* (PAH SHAH).—Cat step. Temps 2-4. A dancer, dressed in the head of a cat, bounds and jumps over obstacles purposely placed. Then he bounds upon a piece of furniture or a table, and does the following steps. Spring in the air and alight on the l.f., bending r. leg (the r. leg should be near l. ankle, the foot on r. side, and the sole of this foot on the r. side), the two hands held in position as a frightened cat. Repeat with the other foot *Another description.*—Stand in 5th right front. Bend both knees (*plié*) and smartly round |the r. leg and throw it to 2nd position, immediately placing l.f. in 5th rear ; repeat as often as needed.

Chat, demi queue du (KER DER SHAH).—Cat's tail. Known also as *demi-promenade*. In square dances. Each person of two opposite couples presents l. hands to partner and goes off obliquely to the right to the opposite side to change places (4 bars). Regain places with demi chaîne anglaise (4 bars).

Cheiroskatiskos.—An ancient Greek dance, so called because it was danced with a basket of flowers in the hand. It was mentioned by Athenée and Pollux.

Chica, *la* (SHE-KA).—Dumb-show, quick 3-4 dance from Cuba, 1495. The dance is a kind of struggle, in which all the strategies of love and the means of triumph are brought into play. Fear, hope, disdain, tenderness, caprice, pleasure, refusal, excitement, passion, ruin, flight, in fact there is a complete love history in this dance, which pourtrays all the dancer has been able to get into his life. The various steps expressing these emotions are infinite, and are executed in jumping, gliding, agitating the loins; the lady holds a handkerchief on her skirt. The gentleman, with pas sautés, advances and retires, imploring her to give him her love.

Chireon Apokope.—Greek dance, done during the carving of meat at feasts. It is known that among the Greeks, the meat was carved while the guests were entertained by singing and dancing.

Chironomie.—Ancient Greek war dance, often mistaken for the Pyrrhic, although it differs in many respects. It had as much success with the Romans as with the Greeks. Xenophon and Hippocrates wrote long eulogies on it. Apulee, Julius Pollux, and Athenée exalted the dancers of this dance. It consisted of a series of gestures with the arms and hands, representing movements which would happen in the thick of battle. Ultimately, its original character became modified, and, science assisting, graceful and slower gestures effected the style. It was staged in the Roman theatres, and Juvenal, in his Sixth Satire, vaunts the success of Bathylle dancing the Chironomie before the Roman ladies. The Greek word "*Chironomie*" is translated as "*danse des mains.*"

Chorégraphy (KORÉGRAFI).—As its Greek name indicates, this means to write out or describe a dance, that is to say, to put down by writings and drawings the different steps of a dance. Musicians write their notes with signs marked on four lines, chorégraphy indicates the steps by a line showing the direction of the dancers, and secondly, whether they move to the right or left. Signs in music are called notes, in dancing they are called steps. The first essays on chorégraphy were written by Jean Tabourot, under the *nom de plume* of "Thoinot-Arbeau," and published in 1588. These essays have not, properly speaking, a chorégraphic character, because they contain no signs. These are supplemented by written descriptions. We must pass on from 1588 to 1707 and 1713 to find the chorégraphic language and writing, in the works of Feuillet and Desaix. These dance-masters published the first chorégraphical treatise, in which they inserted the dance theories. Some years later the best and most complete work was that of Margny, which is a real dictionary of dance terms, giving all the signs employed and their definitions. This book is a correct dictionary of all the chorégraphical art. It is most interesting from the point of view of ancient menuets and dances which can easily be translated, even the most complicated steps. If one is not initiated in the signs which describe dancing, it is only necessary to refer to the sign in Margny's Dictionary to find the description. Thus the feet are described as o— r.f., —o l.f.; the feet together being —oo—. In more modern times, Sultzer, Roller, Carlo Blasis, Arthur de St. Léon, Bernard Klemm, and Friedrich Albert Zorn invented systems of dance writing (chorégraphy).

Choréion (KORAYON).—Meursius, in his index of ancient dances simply mentions this dance without indicating the class to which it belongs, the word, however, implies a dance composed of steps united to words.

Choréios (KORAYOS).—Choir of dancers. Name given to an ancient troupe of dancers, accompanied by singers. The remotest mention of the name dates from the time of Moses, after the passage across the Red Sea. Two large choirs were assembled by him, one composed of men, presided over by him, the other of women, led by his sister, Miriam. The two choirs, with tambourines, danced and sang the canticle "Cantæmus Domino." In the early churches a space was reserved at the end of the building which was called the "chœur." The choir itself was represented by the dancers or the ballet, examples of which were the celebrated choirs established by Pylades in Rome. It is principally to the early Roman theatres that we owe the choirs of dancers; in the Greek choirs, dancing alone was not included. Pylades, who was an artist and dancer, as ingenious as he was clever, introduced these choirs of singers and dancers to add to the brilliancy and effect at the theatre. He harmonized the steps with words and gestures, and was the creator of great scenic representations. He was the first who discovered the importance and the art of costuming. In modern days, "coryphée" is employed as the term for the dancer, "choir" being understood as a body of singers or choristers.

Chute (SHOOT).—A fall. After a jump (*sauter*), one naturally falls to the ground on the feet, either on the sole, heel, ball or point. The fall step is *tombé*. If it is intentionally made audible, it is a *chute*.

Cinq Pas—*Five Pas*. In olden times it was said that five movements could be originated with the help of the knees, ankles, and feet. Modern dance-teachers have, however, increased the number to eight. They demonstrate on a simple basis every action the legs can perform in dancing. The terms are the fundamental technical terms employed in dancing :—

1. *DROIT; in a straight line forward or backward.*
2. *OUVERT; open sideways - right or left.*
3. *ROND; in a circle* (analogous with pas de basque).
4. *TORTILLÉ; winding or twisting.*
5. *GLISSÉ; gliding the foot on the ground.*
6. *SAUTÉ et RETOMBÉ; jumping or springing and the naturally accompanying alighting on the feet.*
7. *TOURNÉ; turning.*
8. *BATTU; beating one foot against the other.*

Circassian Circle.—An unlimited number of persons can join in this dance, which consists of any figure adapted from a square dance. Usually it is the first figure of the Caledonians. The couples are arranged in a large circle round the room, each two couples facing each other. All commence simultaneously and dance first figure of Caledonians till the end of the ladies' chain. Then turn partner in place (4 bars) and chassez to next facing couple (4 bars). Repeat the whole *ad lib.*

Ciseaux *or* **Sissonne** (SEE-SO, SISSONN) temps and pas.—R. Voss in his " Dictionary of Dances," mentions the Sissonne as the name of a Provençal dance performed in 1565, at a festival of the French Court, but no description is given. This scissor step consists of two temps or syllables. If during the first temps, the weight rests on both feet, but on the second temps is supported on only one, it is a *step* or *pas* (*pas de sissonne*). But, if the weight remains on the same support during both syllables, it is a *temps de sissonne.* The step is thus described by Zorn:—" Prepare by standing with l.f. in 2nd elevation. (1) during a light jump on r.f., the l.f. is put down into 5th rear, ball position, both knees bent. (2) jump and fall back on one foot only, while the other foot is quickly raised to 2nd elevation, preparatory for the next step. If the stepping foot is put down in front, it is *pas de ciseaux dessus;* if to the rear or under crossed, it is *pas de ciseaux dessous."* It can also be made *alternatif.* PAS DE CISEAUX DOUBLE, is thus described by Bernard Klemm in his "Catechism of the Art of Dancing." " In place. Preparation, 5th r.f. forward. (1) bend knees and jump on both feet, alighting in 5th point position. (2) jump again, falling on l.f., while r.f. is stretched to 2nd elevation until (3) it falls back again into the 5th, either dessus or dessous. This step occurs in the English Sailor's Hornpipe." CISEAUX for jigs, etc., (turning to the right). Stand in 1st position (1) turn on sole of r.f. so that the foot is turned in, at the same time, turn on l. heel inward. The heels will now be open, and the toes touching. (2) turn on r. heel and l. sole, opening the r. point and shutting l. heel, finishing in 1st position. Repeat. CISEAUX forward and to rear. The heels united, and the points open. (1) close the points and open the heels in advancing. (2) shut the heels and open the points. Continue the whole, *ad libitum.*

Cliquetis.—A dance peculiar to the Romans, composed by Romulus who taught it to his warriors. They, in full armour, sprang roughly and ran in imitation of savages.

Closed Positions.—The 1st, 3rd and 5th positions.

Coin (KWAHN) or À COIN.—Corner or angle. Commonly known in square dances as the "corner" lady or gentleman, that is, the lady standing at the gentleman's l. side, and the gentleman standing at the lady's r. Example, tour à coin = turn corners (in 1st figure of Lancers).

Comus.—The composer of the festal dances of the Greeks and Romans.

Contredanse (CORNTR-DAHNS).—Originally an English country dance ; since 1710, introduced in France, it consists of various figures, generally performed by four couples, six couples (double sides) or eight couples (a double set). Now known as the Quadrilles (*see* Quadrilles). Succeeding the Menuets, the contredanses were full of gaiety, and heralded a style of dancing which was quicker and more sprightly. Chaines, grands ronds and balancés were the principal features, but they were regulated by the leader of the dance, and were not fixed or "set" as in the modern quadrilles, which are always the same. There was an infinite number of steps, but the principal were:—Chassés, la Jalousie, les Cotillon and la Mariée. Trénitz was a fervent performer of the dance, and one figure bears his name. Since 1830, the Contredanse has gone through many changes in its general character. Primitively gay, bright and frivolous, it has become so sad and apathetic that it can scarcely be reconciled with the old gaiety. The origin of the word Contredanse is *contra saltare* or *danser contre*, dancing facing each other. In 1748, Rameau introduced the first into his ballets. Diderot's " Encyclopædia" commits an error by including contredanses among dances executed by one couple only. We find no trace of any dance bearing this name, executed by one couple, in any other work, not even in the antique Dictionary by Trévoux.

CONTREDANSE.—Some primitive figures:—

L'AURORE.—(1) One couple chassé to side couple and two balancés with side couple. (2) Turn with both hands to place. Repeat for the other three couples. (3) lady dance solo during eight bars. (4) same lady cross to vis-a-vis gentleman, turn, recross, and balancé first with r. hand then l. hand, then a turn with both hands. (5) grand circle.

LA FOLATRE.—(1) demi chaîne Anglaise. (2) balancé. (3) demi chaîne Anglaise. (4) balancé. (5) four gentlemen en avant (advance). (6) four ladies en avant. (7) chassé-croisez with partner and places. (8) ladies chain. (9) advance with chassés to the sides, balancé, rond and return to places. (10) chassé avant-quatre. (11) all balancé and turn with both hands. Repeat.

LE CALIFE.—(1) one gentleman en avant et en arriére. (2) vis-a-vis lady repeat. (3) Repeat for all the others. (4) same gentleman and the three ladies advance. Turn by the hands to places. (5) gentleman balancé with partner, turn by hands. (6) gentleman chassé sideward, balancé turn with hands with side lady, and return to place; repeat this with the other three ladies. (7) same gentleman, balancé with partner, turn with both hands, then grand circle. Repeat for the other dancers.

LES BACCHANTES.—(1) all chassé, balancé, and return to places. (2) all, the same in a cross and grand circle. (3) avant-quatre. (4) chaîne Anglaise. (5) balancé. (6) turn with both hands. (7) four ladies, solo each one in turn for four bars. (8) same for the gentleman. (9) all chassé forward and backward. (10) all chassé croisé.

LA TRIOMPHANTE.—(1) chaîne Anglaise two couples. (2) other two couples repeat. (3) the gentlemen, each in turn, in an avant-deux, balancé and turn by the hands; the lady turns for two bars only, then, abandoning the gentleman, she advances to centre, executes four bars solo, and returns to place. (4) the last gentleman and partner turn with both hands. (5) the lady advance to centre and solo eight bars. (6) all the gentlemen advance, join hands, and make a circle round the lady; the lady disengages herself, and all return to places. Repeat for the other couples.

Other figures are LE PETIT MAITRE, LA JALOUSE, LA VIRGINIE, etc.

Contrepas (CORNTR-PAH).—A Catalan dance. Very much danced in Spain at Fêtes Champêtres. The dancers are placed in a circle, hands joined—except the leader who shows the dance. The grave music and the varied movements sideways, forward, backward, parting and drawing together, gives the dancers a melancholy aspect. Women are excluded from this dance.

Contrepoids (CONTR-PWOI).—Equilibrium or equipoise. All dancers must observe this as attentively as centre of gravity. In round dances, gentlemen specially must observe it to guide his partner properly ; he is responsible for her in all round dances. Some women are not only heavier than others, but they are more difficult to lead. Instead of following the men's movements, they stiffen themselves from the waist and even push away his r. arm. If he is not in complete possession of his balance or equipoise he will be unable to lead or "steer" his partner. He must keep his balance solidly to maintain the equilibrium of both. It is evident that for the lady it is less important, yet, she should possess lightness and adaptability to give her partner assurance and confidence.

Contretemps (KORNTR-TAHM).—Means "an accident." In music it means "out of time" or "syncopation." A pas composed of several movements and much employed in the dances of the 17th and 18th centuries. In the "Encyclopædia" of d'Alembert this step is called the "*cloche-pied*." Afterwards contretemps were invented for the Gavotte and Chaconne, and danced *en avant* thus :—With l f. in front 4th position, bend l. knee. Hop and simultaneously pass r.f. to 4th front. The contretemps of the Chaconne were open, that is to the side thus :—L.f. is forward supporting the weight. Hop on l.f. and degagé r.f. to 2nd position, and l.f. immediately crosses to 5th rear. CONTRETEMPS DESSUS.— The leg is crossed first to rear then in front in time to the music. CONTRETEMPS DESSUS ET DESSOUS.—The movements of the feet are the same, crossing the feet but doubling the time, performing two contretemps in the same time. CONTRETEMPS BATTUS.—In executing the contretemps beat one leg against the other. This battement can also be executed in turning and produces a brilliant effect in stage dancing. DEMI-CONTRETEMPS.—Stand in 2nd elevation. The free leg is carried to a closed position, then an open one and touches the supporting leg either rear and before, or before and rear, but does not receive the weight.

Coquette, *pas de* (KOKET).—Two bars 2-4 time. (1) glissade l.f (2) draw r f. up to l.f. (3-4) repeat. (5 to 8) pas de polka with l.f. Repeat with r.f. (2 bars).

Coranto or **Courante.** (*See* Courante).

Corbeille (KOR-BY-E).—A basket. Name given to various figures in Square dances and Cotillons. In the Cotillon it is formed thus :— Three gentlemen are placed in a line with their partners in the centre of the ballroom ; they advance and retire ; the two gentlemen placed at the left and right of the centre one pass beneath the arms of the ladies to the right and left of the line of ladies. The two gentlemen join hands behind the centre lady, the two ladies join hands behind the centre gentlemen. This "basket" is converted into a circle without releasing hands and the circle moves round to the left. The dancers raise their arms and break the circle by releasing hands.

Cordace or **Cordax.**—Greek theatrical eccentric dance. Vivacity, eccentricity and fury characterise it.

Corde, *pas de la* (DE LA MATELOTTE).—The dancer imitating (with hands and feet) a sailor climbing up a rope. Jump on l.f. lifting r. knee high, then pass r. toe in front of l., legs crossed and the toes pointed to the ground and together. Repeat, jumping on r.f.

Corkscrew. (*See* Tire-bouchon).

Coronatia.—Dance by R. M. Crompton.

Corps (KORE).—The body. *Tour de corps.* The turn or movements of the body. (*See* tour de corps).

Cosaques (KO-SAHK).—Theatrical dance by Zorn. Tempo 2-4. When this dance is executed by a gentleman and a lady, as a dance, as is often the case in Russia, the spectators place themselves round the dancers. The changes, the movements and the figures are very arbitrary according to the ability of the dancers and the amount of space they have at their disposition. If the dance is done in a drawing-room, space permitting, each part of 8 bars of music can be repeated. Danced in the theatre, there are 4 bars for the introduction and entry of the dancers ; danced in the ballroom, these are used for the salute. During the final coda the dancers leave the ballroom.

Prelude.—4 bars, gentleman and lady enter at the same time, lady from the right, gentleman from the left, by four coupés russes steps (these are glissés and frappés), lady with the l.f., gentleman with r.f.

First part.—1st bar, gentleman's step. During the first half of the 1st bar he does a pas de basque to the right, in doing a half of a turn to the right thus he has nearly turned his back to the audience. During the second half of the 1st bar he jumps on the l.f. and raises himself, the r.f. backwards at the height of the calf. He lifts the r. arm and places his l. hand on his hip. 2nd bar, three pas frappés in place, commence after a little spring on the l.f. from the r.f. in the 3rd position on the ground. After three steps the l.f. beats in the 3rd position in front of the r.f., and the r.f. beats in the 3rd position behind the l.f. Weight of the body on the r.f. and the l.f. prepares to do the same steps during the 3rd and 4th bars. 3rd and 4th bars, this time half-circle to the left, r. arm lifted, l. hand on the hip. 5th—8th bars, repetition of the four preceding bars ; during these 8 bars make a half-turn. 8th—16th bar, repetition of the steps of preceding 8 bars ; the lady makes the same steps with the other foot.

Second Part.—Solo by the gentleman. 1st position, arms crossed in front of the chest. The steps are made en avant during the 8 first bars, and en arrière during the 8 last bars. 1st bar, (1) bend both knees, turned outwards ; (2) straighten knees, spring and tomber (*fall*) in 2nd position on the heels, the length of a foot en avant.

2nd—6th bars, repetition of 1st bar five times. 7th bar. (1) bend the knees; (2) jump and écarté *(throw the legs wide)*, tomber on the heels. 8th bar, three pas frappés in place in the 3rd position starting with l.f. behind the r., backs of the hands on the hips. 9th bar, (1) bend l. knee and beat at same time, with the r.f. in the 2nd position stretched out ; (2) then the weight of the body on the r.f., and lift the l.f. en arrière (at the height of the calf). 10th bar, repeat the movements of the 9th bar commencing with the other foot. 11th and 12th bars, repeat the movements of 9th and 10th bars. 13th, 14th and 15th bars, repeat steps of 10th, 11th and 12th bars. 16th bar, three pas frappés, commence with l.f. behind in the 3rd position.

Third Part.—Solo by the lady. Position, l.f. in 3rd position on the toe, r. hand on the hip. The movements executed during the 2 first bars, to the left, en avant, during 3rd and 4th bars, to the right, en avant (zig-zag forward). 1st bar, spring on r.f., at same time fouetté with l.f. in the 2nd and 3rd elevations dessus (beneath) (fouetté, jump from the 2nd to 3rd elevations) ; (2) the same but fouetté with r.f. in the 2nd and 3rd elevation dessous (above). 2nd bar, same movement as the 1st bar, the spring during 1st and 2nd eighths of the bar. During 2nd beat jeté on the l.f. crossing r.f. in front of l f. en l'air, between the 2nd and 4th positions. 3rd—8th bars, repeat these movements alternate feet. 9th bar, repeat en arrière. 10th, 11th and 12th bars. these movements are repeated changing the foot for each bar. 13th - 16th bars, complete a half-turn to the right, executing the same steps as from 9th to 12th bars

Fourth Part.—Solo by the gentleman. 1st—6th bars, six steps as follows: bend both legs, stretch out r. leg in the 2nd position, widened (to more than a foot's distance) on the toe, heel outwards. Second time on the heel, then the contrary and so on, moving en avant during each bar the length of one foot. 7th bar, bend as far as the thigh, and one spring from this 1st position. 8th bar, three pas frappés in 3rd position, l.f., r.f., l.f. 9th bar, (1) a little spring on the l.f. and a frappé on the flat with r.f. in 5th position above, changing the weight of the body on to this foot (degagé), and making a little spring on the r.f., lifting the l. en l'air at the height of the knee en arrière ; (2) frappé with l f. in 5th position above and degagé, a little spring at once on the l.f., and lift the r.f. en l'air three-fourths above the ground en arrière. 10th bar, the last spring on l.f., prepare the start of the step of this bar. 11th bar, one strong frappé with the r.f., and dégagé to perform a big spring during the 2nd beat. 12th bar, frappé the soles of the feet en l'air (tiré right). 13th, 14th and 15th bars, repeat the movements of 1st bar ; during the 15th bar accomplish a turn of the body to the right. 16th bar, three pas frappés.

Remark.—If the dancer is not tired he should repeat the frappés of the soles during the last 2 bars.

Part Five.—Second solo by the lady. During the 2 first bars zig-zag to the left. 1st bar, jeté with l.f. to the l., and pas bourré, 2nd bar, repeat. 3rd bar, pas de basque making a complete turn (pirouette basque) to the left ; during this movement the arms describe a grand circle. 4th bar, three pas frappés. 5th—8th bars, repeat the 4 bars to the right. 9th bar, preparation, 5th position r.f. beneath ; direction en arrière. (1) spring with half-circle to the right and changement de pieds (changement de pieds making half turn to the right). (2) the l.f., which is forward, turn the point inwards and outward (tortillé). 10th bar, repeat with the other foot, completing half turn to the left. 11th--16th bars, repeat same three times.

Part Six.—Solo by the gentleman. 1st bar, en avant; plier the thigh, spring and fall in the 2nd position, the heels apart. 2nd bar, the same, tomber on the toes, tourné inwards. 3rd bar, as the 1st bar. 4th bar, like the 2nd and the 1st, execute both rapidly during one bar. 5th—7th bars, equal to the 2nd—4th bars. 8th bar, plier to the ground, spring and fall in 5th position, l.f. forward. 9th bar (1) spring, écarté, making half turn in the air to the left, falling in the 5th position. (2) turn the r.f. rapidly inwards and outwards and assemblé in 5th position. 10th—16th bars, repetition of steps of the 9th bar.

Part Seven.—Solo by the lady. 1st bar, zig-zag, en avant, to the left. (1) spring on r.f., meanwhile place the tip of the l.f. in the 2nd position en dehors; lift the r. hand, during this movement describing a circle en dedans. (2) spring on l.f., the heel of the l.f. in the 2nd position, stretching the knee in the 2nd position. 2nd and 3rd bars, repeat. 4th bar, one jeté to the left and two frappés changés (with r. and l.) 5th—8th bars, repeat 4th bar four times. 9th and 10th bars, zig zag, en arrière, to the left; four pas chassés executed feet parallel, beating the heels, backs of the hands on the hips. 11th and 12th bars, frapper the heels five times, describing grand circles, finishing, the backs of the hands on the hips. 13th—16th bars, repeat movements of 11th and 12th bars twice.

Part Eight.—Solo by the gentleman. 1st—8th bars, for each bar bend nearly to the ground, spring and fall on one of the feet in 4th position en avant, on the heel the other on the toe. Commence with r.f. and change the foot for each bar. 9th bar, zig-zag en arrière, to the right, during 9th and 10th bars; one chassé step to the right. 10th bar, bend to the ground, and fall in the 2nd position on the heels, making a grand circle to the right. 11th and 12th bars, pas de coq en arrière and frapper the soles of the feet (*see* 4th, 9th, and 11th bars). 13th to 16th bars, same as 9th and 12th bars, commencing with l.f., zig-zag to the left and en arrière.

Part Nine.—Opposite way—16 bars.

Part Ten.—Gentleman and lady together, at the end of the scene or of the ballroom. Gentleman and lady join r. hands, also l. hands, crossed in front, the couple side by side. 1st to 8th bars (1) pas de basque to the right, making half turn and raising the arms. (2) jump on the l.f., lifting the r.f. en arrière, like the movements of 1 and 9, but zig-zag, to the right and left, en avant. One of these steps is done during each of the 8 bars. 9th and 10th bars, two coupés, r.f. en avant during each of these 2 bars. 11th and 12th bars, salute (reverence) to the public. 13th, 14th, 15th, and 16th bars, turn towards each other with reciprocal reverence.

Cosaque Russe.—Time 2-4, danced by two people (or four). *1st step,* échappé by four attitudes, turning each time you take it up, each time with a step forward. *2nd step,* bourrée en avant and en arrière. *3rd step,* three jétés, turning to the side, and with each foot,

4th step, écart Chinois, three changement de pieds, brisé, entrechat.
5th step, grand écart, three changement de pieds, brisé, entrechat.
6th step, entrechat, attitude, ailes de pigeon, brisé, entrechat, one
turn to the right, one turn to left, brisé, entrechat. 7th step, demi-
pas Russe en avant, glissade en arrière, brisé, ailes de pigeon, brisé,
entrechat. 8th step, brisé with each foot, two entrechat (twice),
sissonne Anglaise to the left. 9th step, ballonné to the side, jété en
arrière, brisé, entrechat to the right, and to the left. 10th step, pas
Russe en avant, déboîté en arrière. 11th step, ailes de pigeon
coupés three times, brisé, entrechat ; do this step a second time.
12th step, d'été twice. Then do the half only, sink on the knees,
raise yourself with an entrechat. 13th step, chassé ouvert en
avant, one turn to the right, chassé ouvert, two turns, and jété en
tournant.

Cotillon (COT-E-YON), often mis-spelled *Cottillion.*—In the 18th century
the Cotillon was only a simple figure of the contredanse, imitating a
popular dance, when the dancers sang a chorus as they danced. There
were two kinds of Cotillons. Le Grand and Le Petit. Both were composed of menuet figures, with which were intermingled, contretemps,
chassés, entrechats, and even cabrioles. Le Grand was danced by
any number, Le Petit by two. In 1830, round dances, which were the
rage, were introduced into it. The art of conducting a Cotillon is
quite a science, and requires experience. The conductor must be gay,
active, good tempered, and possessed of enough moral authority to
make himself obeyed by the other dancers. He must be equally inter-
ested in all, and show no favour. The choice of figures is of two kinds,
the first distinctly classical, as le miroir (mirror), l'eventail (fan), le
berceau (the cradle), les drapeaux (the flags), la clef des cœurs (key
of hearts), la mer agiteé (the agitated sea). The second is for those
who like innovations, such as historical entries, a village wedding, a
pavane, even a circus attended by its tumblers, clowns and animals.
The success of the Cotillon depends on its accessories and their
originality. Beautiful and valuable presents, such as jewels, cigarette
cases and holders, pins, watches, etc., are often given. The French
Cotillons are more modest, the prizes being charming but of no value,
save for the honour of winning them, and as souvenirs. The numbers of accessories cannot be exactly estimated, but three at least
must be reckoned for each dancer. The Cotillon is a dance which
obeys no fixed rules. It should last from one to three hours, and
end with a procession before the host and hostess.

Guide to the Cotillon.—The Cotillon should be conducted
by a Master of the Ceremonies and a young girl, or by a couple
who are good dancers and intelligent leaders, and know how to
choose figures which will interest and amuse the society in which
they find themselves. These are called the "leaders," and they are
responsible for all favours and accessories. The lady distributes
favours, presents, and accessories to the gentlemen, and she invites
them to join in the figures. The gentleman does the same
for the ladies. He presents the lady with the favour as he
solicits his dance, the ladies do *vice versa.* The leaders request all
the couples to sit round the ballroom, while they remain in the
centre. They number each couple No. 1, 2, etc., and command the
band to play a waltz, during which they promenade round the ballroom, followed by all the other couples to the right. Then the

CO PRONOUNCING DICTIONARY OF

leaders commence to waltz, all the couples following once round the ballroom. He then either taps a tambourine or claps his hands, and each couple returns to place. This signal is always the same to commence or terminate the figures. When the ice is broken after the promenade and waltz, the ladies place themselves back to back in the centre of the ballroom, the gentlemen forming a huge circle around them. At a signal from the leader the gentlemen stop, clasp the lady opposite them, and resume the waltz. At another sign from the leader, the ladies form a circle around the gentlemen, who are back to back, and they proceed the same way as before. Another figure which is a useful start to the Cotillon is the *Flirt-dance* or *Introductory Figure*. Each couple executes a promenade, followed by a waltz. At a signal from leader, all change partners for a new promenade and waltz. At another signal, say after sixty-four bars, the couples rejoin as at first. This can be repeated *ad lib*, but always returning to original partner after each change of ladies. Then the leading couple place themselves in the middle of the ballroom. The gentleman explains clearly and concisely, though gaily, each figure as it starts. Some figures are simple, others complicated, so they must be cleverly alternated. It is on the gaiety of the leaders and the attention of the dancers, that the success of the Cotillon depends. There are, speaking roughly, three kinds of Cotillons. *The first*, danced in very strict society, consisting of a few classical figures, without accessories, practised months in advance by some twenty couples, each retaining their own partners. *The second* is the more general. Gaiety rejuvenates the classical figures, and everybody is at his or her ease. This Cotillon includes several accessories and souvenirs. It is conducted by a leader, who takes a turn with each of the dancers. *The third* is a medley, and often too mixed to be pleasant, being merely a parody of the Society Cotillon. The leader—often a novice—contents himself with repeating the figures, showing partiality, and annexing the best accessories. The guests, victims of boredom, are in the company of strangers, who have purchased tickets. It is to be hoped the last kind will be discouraged, as they are a travesty on good society and good form. Thousands of figures can be invented by the leaders, but we give a few as examples:—

AIGUILLES, *les*.—A pincushion with several tapestry needles and ends of wool is presented to a lady. Two gentlemen try to thread the needles, he who is quickest, waltzes with the lady. The pincushion is passed to another lady and the same thing continues.

AILES, *les*.—Wings. Two wings of gauze are pinned to the shoulders of the leading lady. While she dances with her partner, two gentlemen armed with huge cardboard scissors, follow her, seeking to clip her wings. The one who succeeds, dances with her.

ALLER ET LE RETOUR.—Go and return. The leaders form a file of alternating ladies and gentlemen. Followed by his partner and the rest of the file, he winds in and out in various fantasies about the room.

ALLUMETTES.—Matches. A lady distributes matches to all the gentlemen. The one who retains his longest alight, dances with the lady.

AVANT-TROIS, *l'.*—Three advance.—The gentleman leader places himself between two ladies. The lady leader between two gentlemen. The six dancers advance and retire once. Gentlemen accompanying the leading lady raise their arms, and the two ladies who accompany leading gentlemen pass under them without releasing hands. The dancers so placed, turn, then replace themselves in two lines, facing each other. They move forward and backward, terminating with a waltz.

BALAI, *le.*—Broom. Two gentlemen are presented to a lady, who holds a broom. She gives the broom to one of the two gentlemen who dances with it, while she dances herself with the other gentleman.

BALLE EN L'AIR.—Ball in the air. Balls are distributed to the ladies, who throw them among the gentlemen. He who brings back the ball to its possessor, dances with her.

BANDEAU LE BAND.—The lady leader points out a gentleman, who is blindfolded, and conducts him in front of a seated couple. "With whom do you desire to dance," demands the lady. The blindfolded man points. If he points to the gentleman, the couple dance together. He then points in another direction, and if he points to the lady, she dances with him, and her partner is blindfolded.

CHAISES, *les.*—Chairs. Several chairs are placed in the centre of the ballroom, on which gentlemen are seated. All the couples waltz in and out the chairs. If a couple touches a chair, the two gentlemen change places.

CHARIVARI INSTRUMENTAL, *le.*—Discordant Instruments. Musical instruments in cardboard are distributed to all the dancers, who form a large circle, the leading lady in the centre. At a signal from her, everybody begins to play. She dances in the centre with the gentleman who makes most hubbub, whilst the others continue the uproar. General waltz.

CHAT ET LA SOURIS, *le.*—Cat and mouse. Ladies form a grand circle, hands joined, arms uplifted. One lady, chosen by the conductor, passes running beneath the arms of all the ladies, pursued by a gentleman following the same route. When he has caught her, they waltz in centre of circle, whilst the same thing is repeated about ten times. General waltz.

CLOCHE-PIED.—Hopping. All gentlemen, with one leg elevated, hop on the other foot. Like this they pursue the ladies. Directly they catch one, the pair waltz.

COIFFEURS, *les.*—Head-dresses. Paper bags are distributed among the dancers. These bags contain head-dresses in paper. Everyone dons the coiffeur contained in his or her bag. At a sign from the leader, each gentleman seeks the lady wearing the same kind of coiffeur as his, and dances with her.

COUPLES CROISÉS.—Two couples move to meet each other. The gentleman executes a tour de main with his vis-a-vis partner and waltzes with her. The figure is repeated and return to partners.

COURSE EN SAC, *la.*—Three gentlemen place themselves in sacks attached to their waists. Jumping, they pursue two ladies, who only allow themselves to be caught by the gentleman with whom she wishes to dance.

DECORATIONS, *les.*—These are distributed to the ladies, who decorate the gentlemen with whom they wish to dance, and thus the couples rapidly form up.

DEFILÉ, *le.*—The gentlemen, lined up on one side, are numbered from 1 upwards. The ladies, on the other side, are numbered in the same way. At a signal from the leader, the lady and gentleman bearing the number 1, dance together down the line. Arrived at the end, they separate, placing themselves at the ends of the lines. Couples 2, 3, 4, etc., repeat the same movement. At a second signal from the leader, all the couples dance at the same time and regain their places.

DRAP, *le.*—This figure should be executed by twenty ladies and twenty-one gentlemen. The leading couple stretch a sheet vertically. Behind this sheet all the ladies hide. They hold up one arm each, so that the fingers appear above the sheet. At a signal from the leader, each gentleman takes a lady's hand. She is his partner. The gentleman remaining partnerless wraps himself in the sheet and dances alone.

DUEL, *le.*—Foils are given by a lady to two gentleman. The duellists salute and place themselves on guard. The lady balances a ring on a string at the end of a wand between them. The one who manages to catch it on his foil, dances with the lady. The figure continues till all the ladies have found a partner.

ECRAN, *l'.*—Screen. A lady is seated in the middle of the ballroom. The leading lady presents two gentlemen to her bearing a screen. She dances with one of them, whilst the other, following them hopping, hides them with a screen.

ETYMOLOGIE, *l'.*—Two gentlemen are presented to a lady, who, armed with a dictionary, gives them words to explain, little used in the language. The one who gives the best analysis of the words becomes the lady's partner.

EVENTAIL, *l'.*—Three chairs are placed in the middle of the ballroom, two facing one way and one the other way. A lady, invited by the leading gentleman, sits in the centre chair, and two gentlemen, invited by the leading lady, sit on the two others. The lady chooses one to dance with, giving her fan to the other, who should follow the couple, bostonning, and fanning them during the dance.

FANDANGO, *le.*—Four gentlemen place themselves with one knee on the ground. Four ladies execute the double ladies' chain in the centre, turning round the gentleman nearest to them. A general waltz terminates it. The double chain which characterises it, and is also known by the name Moulinet, is executed several times. At a signal from the leader, the gentleman dances with the lady who turns round him.

FARANDOLE, *la.*—About ten chairs are placed about the ballroom, on which ten people seat themselves. All the other dancers form a chain, which the conductor directs. This chain winds among the chairs, and at a signal from the conductor, it disperses, and each gentleman dances with the lady he holds by the r. hand.

FIL, *le.*—A lady lets a thread trail, several yards in length. The gentleman who catches the end of the thread, dances with the lady.

FINALE, *la.*—All the dancers who have taken part in the cotillon, line up, and salute the mistress of the house in turn. The leading couple, marching at the head, place themselves to the front and a little to one side, after having saluted and joining arms, form an arch, continued by all the couples who pass beneath, executing the same movements.

GRAND MOULINET.—Four couples place themselves en moulinet, under the direction of the leader ; the lady at each extremity invites a gentleman ; he invites a lady, and so on until the moulinet comprises all the dancers. At a signal from the leader the moulinet stops, and each gentleman dances with the lady on his left.

GRAND ROND.—The leading lady forms all the gentlemen into a grand circle. The conductor forms another circle around the gentlemen, comprising all the ladies. At a signal they turn, facing each other, and circle round. At a second signal the circles halt, and the gentleman dances with the lady vis-a-vis.

GRIMACES.—Ten of the gentlemen are placed in a line in the middle of the ballroom. Two ladies face them and choose as their partners the two making the most horrible grimaces. The figure is re-commenced and the most comical attitude is chosen. For a third time the ladies can choose the ones making the most grotesque gestures.

HOULETTE.—Shepherd's crook. The conductor holds a crook in the centre of the ballroom with six ribbons of different colours, and each about eight yards long, attached. Six gentlemen place themselves in all directions, facing the crook and holding the ribbons. During this time the leading lady distributes flags of the same colours as the ribbons to six ladies. The ladies approach the gentlemen holding the ribbons corresponding to their flags, and dance with them. The couples turn in dancing round and round the crook, twisting and untwisting the ribbons.

HUIT, *le.*—Two chairs are placed in the centre of the ballroom. The leaders describe, whilst waltzing, a figure 8 around the two chairs. The other couples imitate them. If any move a chair, the gentleman is out of it, and his place taken by another.

MIROIR.—A lady is seated in the centre of the ballroom holding a mirror in one hand, in the other a handkerchief. The gentlemen file past her at the back of the chair and she regards them in the mirror. If the lady wipes the mirror with her handkerchief, the gentleman moves away. If she allows him to look at her, he becomes her partner.

MOULIN.—Four gentlemen place themselves in the position of the wings of a windmill, joining l. hands and giving the r. hand to their partners. The four ladies invite four gentlemen to take their r. hands. These seize them with their l. hands, and offer in their turn the r. hand to four ladies, and so on. The figure is terminated by a general waltz, each gentleman dancing with the lady to the right.

MUSIQUE, *la leçon de.*—The leader gives an instrument to a lady, to whom various gentlemen are presented. The lady strikes a note and makes them give it a name. The one who answers best dances with her.

Myops.—Short-sighted person. A lady is presented to a gentleman, who must find her, in spite of a pair of black spectacles and his being made to turn round several times.

Names.—The leading lady distributes plain cards to the gentlemen, who write their names on them. The conductor collects the cards in a hat, mixes them up, and distributes them to the ladies. These seek out the gentleman bearing the name written on the card to dance with them.

Notary.—The leader asks a lady, in a whisper, which is the lucky number to place with her name. A number is written, and the gentlemen are invited to guess it. The one guessing aright dances with the lady.

Numbers.—A series of numbers from 1 to 20 are distributed to the ladies by the leader. A duplicate series is distributed to the gentlemen by the leading gentleman. The gentleman seeks his partner by the number corresponding to his.

Ombre Chinoise.—Six big umbrellas, decorated with ribbons, are given to the ladies, and six little ones of corresponding colours to the ladies as favours. At a first signal, ladies and gentlemen follow each other, their umbrellas in evidence. At a second signal they exchange umbrellas, the ladies pin the little favours to their dresses, the gentlemen open the large umbrellas, the couples form up, partners finding each other by the colours, and they dance, each couple beneath an open umbrella.

Papillon.—The ladies are armed with butterflies. These they throw at the gentlemen, and dance with those they hook on to.

Parallèles.—The gentlemen and ladies line themselves up in two parallel lines. The gentleman and lady at the head waltz between the two lines and place themselves at the other end. The other couples do the same in their turn, then the lines execute an avant quatre, do a promenade, and the figure terminates by a general waltz.

Passe, la (pâs).—The leading gentleman forms the ladies into one line, the gentlemen into another. He places himself at the head of the gentlemen, the leading lady places herself at the head of the ladies. The leading lady leads the ladies beneath the arms of the gentlemen, after which they form a line, and the gentlemen pass in their turn beneath the ladies arms, and so on. A waltz terminates the figure.

Pont.—A doorway is decorated with flowers and foliage. A bell and a basket of flowers are hung up. A lady is placed beneath, and the gentlemen file in front of her. When she wishes to accept a gentleman as partner, she rings the bell, when she refuses one, she shakes the basket, and he finds himself covered with flowers.

Prison, la (Prizôn).—All the ladies form a grand circle, galoping round a gentleman, who tries to find an exit. When he escapes, he dances in the centre of the circle with one of the ladies who have allowed him to escape. Another gentleman takes his place.

PROMENADE AVEC CHANGEMENT DE DANSEUSE.--The couples are placed one behind the other. They waltz, following one another round. At a signal from the leader all the gentlemen leave their partners and dance with the lady behind them. The gentleman belonging to the last couple dances with the lady belonging to the first.

Cotillon Waltz.—*See* Waltz Cotillon.

Cou-de-pied (KOO-DE-PEE-AY).—Literally, the neck of the foot: the instep.

Coup de Talon (KOO-DE-TAHLON).—Known also as *pas polonaise*; the striking of the heels as in the Polish Mazurka. *See* Battu.

Coupé (KOO-PAY).—The cutting step. This step is made from an open position, through a closed position, into another position; the one foot virtually cuts the other from its place.· Thus:—From the 4th rear, the r.f. is placed 3rd rear, with degagé, and l.f. is put in 4th forward, all in one beat of music; this is COUPÉ DESSOUS. If the foot commences from 4th forward, assuming 3rd forward while the other foot goes to 4th rear, it is COUPÉ DESSUS. If the cutting is done from the second position, it is PAS COUPÉ LATÉRAL. If, as in the second step of the Mazurka, there is a strong knock of the foot, it is a COUPÉ POUSSÉ. If the foot is put down with a strongly-accented audible beat, it is a COUPÉ FRAPPÉ. Another explanation:—Standing with r.f. in 5th front position, raise l.f. to 4th position en l'air rear; with a light throw (1) allow l.f. to descend to 5th rear, (2) simultaneously raising r.f. forward. DEMI-COUPÉ.—When the first half of the step is executed. Thus:—Bend the knees and strongly push out the leg with degagé.

Couple. - In square dances will imply a gentleman and his partner, as distinguishable from "a pair" (a gentleman and his vis-a-vis).

Courante, *temps de* (KOO-RAHNT) —A slow dance step, borrowed from the *Courante,* a long-forgotten dance. It is executed forward and backward. *Preparation forward*: stand in r.f. 4th front. (1) l.f. is drawn to 5th rear.. (2) then to 2nd elevation. (3) from there it describes 1st position, then 3rd position in front of r.f. (4) and, with a slight bend of both knees and gently stretching again, the l.f. is brought into 4th position, and degagé on it. The backward movement is the same, but in opposite direction.

Courante was an old dance vaguely mentioned by Thoinot-Arbeau (1588). It was slow, with glissés terre à terre. It was executed by one couple only, to slow time, usually people of high degree, who walked with slow side glissades. They were often more particular about their bearing than their grace, and tried to prove their ancient nobility by an exaggerated lofty carriage of the head and bust. The Courante of Louis XIV. was soon forgotten, and more animated dances displaced it. The imperfect theory only remains.

Courante, *la.*— Period 1600. 3-4 tempo. The Courante—Italian, Corrente—(courant de l'eau) was a very popular dance. It was a kind of branle, very graceful in execution. It was performed by three couples with pas glissés, executing passes to the right and left en courant and in changing partners. A gentleman conducts his partner to the extremity of the ballroom, and then withdraws to the other extremity. The other couples do likewise. Then the gentlemen advance in turn, each inviting one of the three ladies to dance, they either accept, or refuse by turning their backs, when he invites another. When the lady accepted, he knelt, thanking her for the favour bestowed. They then danced side by side, making the different passes of the dance with pas courantes and pas courus. *Pas couru* is a quick walk, gliding on the soles without leaving the ground, and moving the head and arms uniformly with the foot.

Courante, *pas.*—In 2-4 tempo, slowly. Glide l.f. to 2nd, obliquely forward (the intermediate 2-4 position). Glide r.f. to 4th forward. Draw l f. up to r.f.; all in two beats. Repeat with other foot en arrière.

Courante, *temps de:* in two movements. Stand 5th, r.f. front. Bend both knees *(plié)*. (1) Glide r f. to 2nd position, on the sole, then lower the heel. Plié again, then rise. Then glide r.f. to 4th forward, and draw l.f. to 1st.

Courbé (KOOR-BAY).—*See* Bras, port de.

Course, *pas de.*—Running step. In walking, both feet must touch the floor once in every step. In running, one foot must always be in the air. Running steps on the balls of the feet are the most graceful. Those on the heels are sometimes seen in national dances.

Cracovienne, or **Krakoviak.**—A popular Polish dance, originated in Cracow, as its name implies, under Sigismund, king of Poland, 1510. Tempo 2-4. It is danced by several couples, who follow each other, turning round in circles, and accompanying themselves with a song. The gentlemen strike their spurred boots together. The art of the dance consists in the execution of the most eccentric movements with the greatest bravado, and without damaging the ladies' dresses. The original part of the dance is its accompaniment by an improvised song. When the dancer has made a series of sounds, which could, with an effort of imagination, be called a tune, the branle recommences, and the dancers repeat in chorus the last improvised refrain. While singing and dancing, the gentleman often interrupts himself to encourage his partner with " Danse ma belle, danse," words which are taken up in chorus by the other dancers.

Cracovienne, *la* —Austrian, 1896. Tempo 2-4. Both commence same foot. He clasps lady with his r. arm, and places l. hand behind his back—the lady places r. hand behind the back.

    Gentleman's step.—(1) glide l.f. to side, raise r.f., making a chassé and jeté with l.f. (1 bar). Repeat with same foot thrice (3 bars). Raise l.f. to side, and beat the heels together en l'air (1 bar). Same to right (1 bar). To the left and right again (2 bars). (2) repeat the eight bars commencing r.f. (3) they separate, dancing round each other, and beating the feet alternately en terre and en l'air (16 bars). (4) recommence.

Cracovienne.—From Berlin 1897. By Zorn and Radermacher. Tempo 2-4. Stand as in Waltz position. The gentleman clasps the lady with his r. arm, and l. hand on the hip. Lady places l. hand on his shoulder, and holds the dress with the r. hand. Both commence r.f. *Preparation:*—Rise on l.f., and raise r.f. into 4th forward elevation.

    FIRST PART.—*First bar* (1) glide r.f. forward, lift l.f. 4th rear elevation, bending the knees. (2) jump on r.f., placing l.f. in 4th front elevation, rising on r.f. as preparation for the next step. *Second bar*, repeat first bar, commencing l.f. *Third bar*, repeat with r.f. (These three movements will be three *pas boiteaux*). *Fourth bar* (1) both jump on the soles with the heels outward. (2) knock the heels smartly together. (This will be *echappé talons en dehors*, and *assemblé avec coup des talons*).

SECOND PART.—Gentleman. *Fourth bar*, bend both knees, l.f. slightly raised (the feet move from 1st to 5th position). *Fifth bar*, spring, rising on r.f., and carrying l.f. to the side. This is done three times round the lady during the 5th, 6th, and 7th bars. *Eighth bar*, tap gently on the floor three times, l.f., r.f., l.f. During bars 5, 6, 7, the lady executes three *pas boiteaux*, thus:—(1) spring on r.f., carrying l.f. between 4th and 5th position forward. (2) step on r.f., raising l.f. On the eighth bar she executes the same three taps as the gentleman. Polka steps may be substituted for the last four bars, or used as a variation.

Croisé-Traversé.—Ladies exchanging places in square dances.

Croix, *pas* (KROO-AH).—Jeté to the right and left, with arms extended in the form of a cross, rise by the flexion of both knees, with feet together, come down with feet apart, then assemblé. Spring as high as possible, throwing the legs apart sideways, and touch the toes with the hands.

Csardas or **Czardas.**—Eight bars 2-4 time. Lady and gentleman stand vis-a-vis; gentleman, arms crossed over the chest; lady, hands on the hips. *First bar*, pas de polka, gentleman to left, lady to right; during this step the gentleman turns the r. shoulder forward, the lady turns l. shoulder, looking at each other. *Second bar* (1) gentleman places r. heel in 4th forward position; lady l. heel. (2) place same foot on the point, heel outward. (3) pause in this position. *Third and Fourth bars*, repeat bars 1 and 2, commencing with other foot. *Fifth and Sixth bars*, take partner, and two pas de mazurka. *Seventh and Eighth bars*, pas de polka, making a *demi-tour* (half turn), and take up position to repeat the whole.

Cubistik.—The Greeks designated, by this general term, one class of dancing. The ancient composers divided their dances into three classes:—(1) Cubistik, (2) Sphéristik, (3) Orchestrik.

Cuisse, *pas* and *temps* (KOO-ISS).—The word means, the thigh. The step is so called because of the particular action of the thigh. *Preparation*:—L.f. in 2nd elevation. Bend r. leg, and l. leg beats audibly with the tip in 2nd position, after which, hop to the right, and the l. is put down again in the 2nd, and drawn audibly to 5th position, either dessus or dessous. When several such are made in the same direction, no degagé (or transfer) is made, and it is therefore a *temps de cuisse*, but when with alternate foot, a degagé must be made, and it is a *pas de cuisse*.

Curétes.—The dance of the Corybantes, of the period of the early Titans. It was executed to the sound of fifes, tambourines and bells. Presumably, it was danced in armour, as we see the actors with bucklers, lances, swords and javelins.

Curtsey.—The lady's form of salutation. *See* Bow. A man never curtseys, but bows in response to the lady. If the gentleman and lady, facing each other, glide r.f. to 2nd position with weight (which is the first step of the bow and curtesy), it will be seen that each has the other on the left, and they therefore *salute each other to the left*, the movements, however, being made to the *right*. *Preparation :—* Face partner, feet in 3rd position.

(1) Glide r.f. to second position, and immediately carry l. back to 4th position, the toes only touching the floor, about fifteen inches separating the feet, with l. knee well bent. The l.f. will really be in the intermediate 1–4 point position—that is, between the 1st and 4th positions. Keep weight on r.f.

(2) Commence to bow, at same time bend both knees outward and sideways, slowly sinking until the l. knee nearly touches the floor. This should be simultaneous with the bending forward of the gentleman.

(3) Degagé on to l.f., and slowly rise into an upright position.

(4) Bring r.f. to 3rd front position. Be careful not to look at the floor during the curtsey.

Cushion Dance.—Corruption from "Kissing Dance"; from "The Dancing Master," seventh edition, 1686, p. 208.—"Joan Sanderson, or The Cushion Dance, a Round Dance. Directions for dancing:— This dance is begun by a single person (either man or woman) who, taking a cushion in his hand, dances about the room, and at the end of the tune he stops and sings, 'This dance it will no farther go.' The musician answers, 'I pray you good Sir, why say you so?' (Man.) 'Because Joan Sanderson will not come to.' (Musician.) 'She must come to, and she shall come to, and she must come whether she will or no.' Then he lays down the cushion before a woman, on which she kneels, and he kisses her, singing, 'Welcom, Joan Sanderson, welcom, welcom, welcom.' Then she rises, takes up the cushion, and both dance singing, 'Prinkum, Prankum, is a fine dance. and shall we go dance it once again, once again, and once again, and shall we go dance it once again.' Then making a stop, the woman sings as before, 'This dance, etc.' (Musician.) 'I pray you, Madam, etc.' (Woman.) 'Because John Sanderson, etc.' (Musician.) 'He must, etc.' And so she lays down the cushion before a man, who, kneeling upon it, salutes her, she singing 'Welcom, John Sanderson, etc.' Then he taking up the cushion, they take hands and dance round, singing as before. And thus they do till the whole company are taken into the ring. And then the cushion is laid before the first man, the woman singing 'This dance, etc.' (as before), only instead of 'come to,' they sing 'go fro'; and instead of 'Welcome, John Sanderson,' they sing 'Farewel, John Sanderson, farewel, farewel'; and so they go out one by one as they came in. Note that the woman is kiss'd by all the men in the ring, at her coming in and going out, and the like of the man by the woman."

Czarine (ZAR-EEN).—Composed as a Waltz in 1856, by the Academy of Dance Teachers in Paris. In spite of the originality of its title, it met with little success in the ballroom. The theory, as published by the Society, is:—"The Czarine is danced to 3-4 time, with a Mazurka movement, and as in waltzing, is done turning to right, reversing, advancing and retiring. It is composed of four steps, one step to a bar, with alternate foot. Gentleman commences l.f.. lady r.f. THE STEP.—*First bar*, pas polonais or temps de talon. (1) assemblé l.f. in front, beating lightly with the heels. (2) glide same foot to side. (3) coupé with r.f., l.f. remaining in the air. *Second bar*, pas russe or de basque. (1) jeté on l.f., r.f. slightly raised. (2) place r.f. on floor, apart, following the direction of the step. (3) draw l.f. up, and push the r.f. by a light beat of the heel, the r.f. remaining raised. *Third and Fourth bars*, holubieck or tour sur place. (1) r.f. to 4th rear. (2) pivot a half-turn on the points, and change the foot. (3) raise r.f. This step should be made with a half-turn. For the next bar repeat the holubieck with the other foot. Repeat the whole. Lady does same with opposite foot. A complete turn will have been made. For the promenade, the holubieck is replaced by two pas russe or pas de basque."

D

Danaï.--An ancient Greek dance, representing the fable. The dance, whilst simulating the carrying off of the Ganymede, left in the soul the most beautiful and tender impression.

Dance.—Movement of the body in harmony with the rhythm of the music, producing expressive motion. Dancing, originally, had not the same meaning as the modern idea. Primitively, it was a rough means of expressing different emotions by gestures, jumps, and turns. All the ancient Greek dances, excepting the Cubistick and Cordace, were executed terre-à-terre. The history of dancing, which is as old as the world itself, offers an unlimited field of research to those who have patience and the courage to work, determined to triumph over the difficulties of the enterprise.

The Ancients divided dancing into three parts: (1) Sacred and Religious, (2) Military, (3) Private and Social.

Zorn says, "(1) Dancing is the expression of pleasure or other sentiment by means of prescribed movement, regulated by music, either imagined or expressed. (2) Its factors are: Position, Movement, Figure, and Measure. (3) Transition from one position to another is accomplished by means of Movements, which are either simple or compound. (4) The line described on the floor by the dancers is the Figure. (5) The division of the movements into periods of a certain duration, to correspond with the music, is called Measure. Simple figures correspond to verses, compound figures to stanzas, and the connection of compound figures or strophes, as in a Quadrille, to an entire poem."

Dancing. (Arguments in favour of).—"The love of motion, and of rhythm in that motion, is innate in the human breast, and no amount of condemnation by well-meaning but short-sighted people can deprive us of that part of our natures. That the influence of rhythm is irresistible is proved by the readiness of hand or foot to spring involuntarily into motion to keep time with a well played piece of music, and also by the unmistakable access of confidence which comes to the most timid 'raw recruit' in a regiment when the drum beat sends the men along with a perfect consonance of movement.

"Whether her children should or should not be taught dancing is a question that confronts every mother, sooner or later. Many people, actuated by the purest and most distinguished of motives, are ceaseless in their censure of this graceful exercise and recreation, because they lose sight of its advantages in their disgust for its frequent abuse by the unrefined. The benefits, both mental and physical, which the young derive from a mastery of the art of dancing are manifold. Children who attend a well conducted dancing school, cannot but be impressed with the gracious politeness exhibited on every side, so that even boys who have previously been rough and careless in their manners are quickly brought to appreciate the beauty of courtesy, and acquire habits of gentle speech and action, that exert a salutary influence as long as they live. Physiologists have for many years regarded dancing as one of the finest of gymnastic exercises, and declare it to be superior to all others in its beneficial effect upon the carriage and manner. Graceful motion is always easy motion, and, therefore, causes much less wear and tear upon the physical machinery than angular and awkward actions.

" It is a mistake to suppose that personal grace is altogether a natural gift, for there have been numerous instances where unusually awkward and ungainly children have been made graceful men and women by careful training. An eminent surgeon, who has devoted the greater part of a long life to the cure and prevention of bodily weakness and deformity in the young, regards dancing as a most necessary branch of physical training, since the preparatory exercises which form part of every dancing lesson stimulate the muscular action, and thus lay a firm foundation for a large degree of health in after years. Angularity and stooping of the shoulders are more frequently the result of habit than of any natural defect or weakness ; and if the attempt to correct these evils is deferred until a child is fourteen or fifteen years of age, the result is rarely successful. Many boys possess a silly notion that it is effeminate to · be graceful ; and their habits of motion and carriage should therefore receive early and effective attention. A child of five is not too young to commence dancing lessons, for at that age every faculty has awakened, and this early cultivation of the powers of observation and concentration are sure to be of mental as well as physical benefit.

Dancing never has a pernicious influence until it is abused. When people dance in hot, crowded rooms, where the atmosphere is unwholesome, where frequent jostlings are unavoidable, and where lack of space renders too close personal contact almost a necessity, it is then that they degrade the beautiful, graceful art, and bring it into ill-repute."

Dancing (Divisions of).—It is divided into two great classes, SOCIAL and THEATRICAL ; the former is done for pleasure, the latter for gain. In social dances the most general are those which are done in " the waltz position," and are called " ROUND" dances. There were also "COLUMN" dances, such as Sir Roger de Coverley, Tempête, etc.; "SQUARE" dances such as Quadrille, Lancers, etc. ; social "SHOW" dances, such as Menuet, Gavotte, Cachuca, Fandango, etc.—any of this class, may, however, be raised to the theatrical dances.

Theatrical danses may be divided into five classes. The lowest degree is (1) THE GROTESQUE ; these are of an unsteady, adventurous type, with movements that are often imposing, but they demand skill rather than grace. (2) THE COMIC are less unsteady. They generally represent the customs, pastimes, and romances of the lower orders. (3) DEMI-CARACTÈRE exemplify affairs of ordinary life by representing on the comic stage a love story or plot, with characters from the common people, and is replete with grace and elegance. (4) SERIOUS: such are of a tragic character, and require the highest degree of skill and elegance. They include *solos, pas de deux*, etc., representing emotions or ideas, and demand the exercise of the entire art. (5) PANTOMIMIC are of the highest order, and represent entire wordless tragedies divided into acts to convey the entire idea. Such dances may be termed Ballets. Most prominent among artistes of this class are Carmago (1710–1770), Mdlle. Sallé (1734), Madeline Guimard (1743–1816), Taglioni (1834), (mother and daughter), Lucille Grahn (1838), Fanny Ellslér, Fanny Cerito (born 1821), Carlotta Grise (1841), Nadeschda Bogdanova, Adeline Genée ; Messrs. Beauchamp (1671), Pécourt (1679), Marcel (1704), Dupret (1717), Gaetan Vestris (1751), and his son Auguste Vestris (1787), Noverre (1777), Gardel (1779), Blasis (1820), Petitpa (1839), A. de St. Léon, etc.

Danse Macabre.—Sombre English dance, 1420. The dancers had skeletons for partners, the music being supplied by instruments made of human bones.

Danseur and **Danseuse.**—Names applied to male and female dancer on the stage.

Déboités (DAY-BWAH-TAY).—Dislocated or disjointed. These steps are made by passing the r.f. behind the l.f., then the l.f. behind the r.f., moving backward or in place.

Début (DAY-BOO).—First appearance, beginning, or entry. Hence, Débutante, an actress or dancer appearing for the first time.

Découverte.—Dance. In use among savages. They attempt the movements of warriors in their warlike excursions in the surprise and discovery of an enemy.

Dédalienne.—Ancient dance. It is depicted on the buckler of Achilles. Lucien wrote a eulogy on it.

Dedans (DAY-DAHN).—Inwardly or forward. It is the opposite of *Dehors*, outwardly or back.

Dégager (DAY-GAH-ZHAY).—To transfer the weight of the body from one foot to the other. No *pas* (step) can be made without this transfer. Movements without the transfer are *temps* or parts of a step.

Dégagement (DAY-GAAZH-MAHN).—The act of transfer.

Dégagé à genoux (DAY-GAH-ZHAY AH ZHEN-OO).—A movement in El Cachucha, in which the dancer is kneeling on one knee, and, raising herself, lowers herself on to the other knee.

Dehors (DAY-OR).—*See* Dedans.

Deinos.—Ancient Greek dance with most solemn movements.

Delienne—Greek sacred dance, consecrated to the fêtes of Delos. Danced by young patrician girls to the flute and lyre. The principal movement was dancing in circles, with joined hands, or holding garlands. The finale was to cover the statue of Venus with the garlands, while the hymn of Diana was sung by the assembly. The girl who was most admired for her dancing was crowned with olive leaves or flowers, and often with precious stones. The Delienne was usually terminated by the young men practising archery, and exercising their skill in piercing a rose attached to the top of a mast.

Démarche (DAY-MARSH).—Gait, walk.

Demi (DRM-MB).—Half. Signifies that a movement or figure is only half done. In square dances, such a figure leads either to the opposite side or from the opposite side back to place.

Dérobé, *pas* (DAY-RO-BAY).—The feet slip, simultaneously, one to the right, the other to the left, or, one forward and the other backward; then they are slipped together again (*assemblé*).

Déroulé or **Détourné** (DAY-ROO-LAY, DAY-TOOR-NAY).—*Déroulé*, to evolute or unroll ; *Détourné* to turn away. Turning to right or left on the sole or points by little steps. Then, *déroulé* or *revolve* the body from the hips, doing the same steps the other way round. The revolving, can also be done on one foot, with the other in the air.

Dervishes.—The most notorious religious fanatics are Whirling or Dancing Dervishes, the Mohammedan priests who spin round on their feet for hours at a stretch without any injurious effect. Their dance is a boring parade, possessed of no merit except the physical endurance of the dancer. Much has been written of the Dervish priest and his ways. Perhaps the most interesting is Clarke's "Voyage in Asia," in which he initiates us into the character and habits of these priests. He says, "As we entered a mosque, we saw twelve or fourteen Dervishes peacefully promenading 'in a circle round the Superior, in a space surrouuded by a balustrade under the dome of the building. Several spectators, divested of their shoes, were outside the balustrade. Two or three musicians were seated Turkish fashion, with tambourines and flutes. First, the dervishes, crossing their arms over their chests and holding their shoulders with each hand, make reverences before the Superior. They then commenced to twirl slowly, then faster, so that their long robes swing round with them and they looked like open umbrellas. As the speed increases, the arms are disengaged from the shoulders and raised gradually to the height of the head. Their eyes are closed as they revolve rapidly. The music, accompanied by voices, animates them, and an old dervish in green vestments walks about quietly among them. The dervishes turn by moving one of their feet, bending the big toes inward at each movement of the body, whilst the other foot keeps an ordinary position. The oldest dervishes appear to execute this dance with very little trouble and fatigue, in spite of the violent agitation of their body, their faces are plunged in what appears a kind of quiet slumber. The youngest and oldest turn with the same agility, but they turn less mechanically than the others. This extraordinary exercise lasts fifteen minutes, and the eyes of the spectators become very weary. At a signal from the Superior, the dervishes stop instantly, and form a circle. All again place their hands on their shoulders, and lower themselves to the ground. They raise themselves and again promenade before their Superior, then, after more salutations, commence twirling again. They persevere until great beads of perspiration run down their faces and bodies on to the floor. At a third signal, the dance concludes."

The Dervish dance is looked on by the Turks as miraculous, and although dancing in couples is interdicted no one would dare to interfere with the priest dancers. These twirling dancers are not the only ones in practice among the Arabs, they execute others known as the "miraculous" dances and "fire" dances. They spring after the manner of our mountebanks, holding bare swords, then, seizing red hot irons, they put them in their mouths, licking them with their tongues. It is supposed that the dervish Ménélaus, according to an interpretation of the Alcoran, was the inventor of the first dervish dance, whilst Hansé, played the flute, Ménélaus, according to the fable, continued pirouetting for fifteen days and nights.

Descendre (DE-SAHN-DR).— To descend. Dancing or walking from the back of the stage down to the footlights. Commonly termed " walking down the stage," which is literally correct ; owing to the slope, one must walk down, while going to the back of the stage, " one walks up."

Dessous (DES-SOO).—Over, or in front.

Dessu (DESSŪ).—Under, or to the rear.

Détourné (DAY-TOOR-NAY).— See Déroulé.

Développé (DAY-VEL-LOPPAY).—To develope. A temps, signifying the slow unfolding of the leg to its full length, whilst placing it in the position demanded. One leg alone supports the body, whilst the other is developed forward, sideward or rear, well turned-out, and at an angle with the supporting leg. Simultaneously with the raising of the leg, the arms should be raised equally in front of the chest, and, after reaching the height of the shoulders, they should separate and form a horizontal line, then lowered to reach the sides at the same moment that the legs are again together.

D'été, pas (DAY-TAY).— Stand r.f. in 5th rear. (1) échappé in 2nd position. (2) with a slight jump on r.f., raise l.f. in rear. (3) l.f. makes a coupé dessous. (4) assemblé r.f. to rear.

Deux (DER).—Two. Any movement in which two persons are occupied, as avant-deux (two advance).

Deux=temps (DER TAHM).—" Two-time." A count of two steps to any dance or dance-music as the " Waltz deau-temps." If the music is in 2-4 temps, and is counted as one beat to the bar, it is commonly known as "half-time "; two bars of 3-4 tempo, counted one to the bar, is deux-temps, as also is a count of two to a bar in 6-8 tempo.

Diane.—Dance instituted among the ancients in honour of Diana. Compan declares it was a sacred dance. Aristophanes one day found all the girls of the town of Carie celebrating, with songs and this dance, the fête of the deity. Before the reformation of Lycurgas, the dances of Diana occasioned the greatest misfortune. Helen, the most beautiful of women, was abducted first by Theseus, then by Parias ; both had been enchanted by her dancing the Diane.

Dionysiac.—This was danced during the festival to Dionysius (Bacchus) ; it was customary in Athens. All the Greek authors were unanimous in the praise of its magnificence and surroundings. Later, the dance degenerated, and gave rise to great scandal owing to the intemperance of the dancers ; this was followed by wild orgies and free licence. It was consequently forbidden to be danced.

Diphodismos. – Greek laconic dance.

Dipodies.—A Spartan dance, in which the feet were used as an offensive weapon.

Dipoliœ.—The Spartans practised this dance during the solemn festivities of the Dipolies.

Dithyrambic —Lyric dances and songs dedicated to Apollo.

Divertissement (DE-VER-TIS-MAHN).—*See* Ballet d'action.

Doliva.—Contredanse of the middle ages ; similar to the Branles, and was danced at village festivals.

Dos-à-dos (DOH-ZA-DOH).—In square dances. Two dancers move round each other, r. shoulder to r. shoulder and back to back, they go either across to opposite side or return to place.

Droit (DROO-AH).—The right ; *à droit,* to the right ; *le main droit,* the right hand, etc.

E

Écart or **Écarté,** *temps* (AY-CARTAY).—Means to spread or disperse ; the movement is also called *spagat,* from the Italian *spalancare,* to open wide or extend Stand in 5th position. During a high jump, throw the legs widely apart and alight on the feet in the preliminary 5th position, or with the other foot in front. ÉCART PAR TERRE is the ground écart, in which the legs are so widened that the body sinks and the legs rest at full length on the floor, one in front the other back. It is commonly known as "splits." GRAND ÉCART is a combination of both movements. Spring in the air, throw the legs wide, and, with the legs widened to their fullest extent, fall to the ground with one leg fully stretched forward, the other backward. This movement should be performed with extreme caution, and requires considerable practice.

Écart Chinois, *pas* (AY-KAR SHE-NWAR). –After bending both knees, rise lightly from the ground, falling with both feet écart in the 2nd position on the heels, and toes turned upward, knees bent, arms forming a square, fingers closed except index or first finger, which points to ceiling.

Écart trépigné (AY-KAR TRA-PE-NAY).—A stamped écart. The changing place on the heels for sailors' hornpipe. Bend the knees and jump on the heels, with the feet écart in 2nd position, the toes pointing to the ceiling, arms crossed in front. From this position advance by beats of the feet and movements of the body. Advance and retreat, the feet remaining in the same position.

Échappé or **Sailli,** *temps* (AY-SHAHP-PAY). To escape. The step consists of a spring with an opening of both feet. From the 5th or 3rd position spring upward and alight with both feet in the 2nd ball position.

Ekateris.—In Greek dances, the clapping of hands without any movement of the feet. Athene describes it as dancing with the hands.

Eklatismos.—Aristophanes mentions this dance as one peculiar to the women, who raised their heels above the height of the shoulders.

Eleusis.—The mysteries of Eleusis were favoured by the Greeks, The festivals consecrated to Ceres and her daughter Prosperine, which were celebrated in the vale of Eleusis, continued for nine days. The first four days were devoted to sacrifices, and on the evening of the fourth day a procession took place, in which a basket on a chariot, drawn by four oxen, figured prominently. The procession was composed of a number of Athenians, carrying baskets covered with purple veils, and containing the objects required for the ceremony. The statue of the deity, crowned with a wreath of myrtle and a lighted torch in the hand, was carried in front of the procession. Following, was a huge procession of women, the number often reaching thirty thousand. At a blast of trumpets, choirs, singers, and dancers expressed the greatest joy. The Eleuses represented a kind of grand moving ballet.

Elevations.—Raisings. The movements by which the body is raised from the floor. They can be made with either or both feet.

Elever and **s'Elever.**—*See* Abaissements.

Élevé, Élever (AIL-VAY).—Means to raise, and refers to the supporting leg, or raising the body. A *temps élevé* is rising on one foot while the other foot does some other movement. A *pas élevé* is a rising step.

Emboiter, pas emboité (PAH-ZAHM-BWAHT-AY).—To fit in; to join. Step movements from a closed into other closed positions, made through placing the feet alternately side by side. *Example:*—From 3rd or 5th position, r.f. in front. The l.f., gliding sideways, passes close to the heel of r.f., and takes the 5th front position. In the same way, the r.f. moves into front 5th position; these are *en avant* or *dessus*. For *pas emboité dessous* or *en arrière*, place the foot to 5th rear ; these are sometimes termed *déboiter*.

En Avant (AHN AH-VAHN).—To advance or forward. *See* Avant.

En Arrière (AHN AH-RE-AIR).—To retire, or rear. *See* Avant.

En avant et en arrière.—To advance and retire.

Enchainement (AHN-SHAYN-MAHN).—The arrangement or combination of steps into a dance or dance figure.

En dedans.—Inward.

En dehors.—Outward.

En haut (AHN-O).—Raised. High up.

En l'air (AHN-LAIR).—In the air. All elevations of the feet and balancing positions are en l'air.

Enlevé (AHN-LEVAY).—Lifting the heels whilst stretching the instep. The term is used instead of *élevé*.

En passant (AHN PAHSSAN).—In passing. Usually a step employed in which one or more persons pass in front or rear of other persons who move in a contrary direction.

En terre (AHN-TAIR).—On the ground. The opposite of en l'air. Any movement of the foot on the floor is said to be *en terre*.

Entrechat (AHNTER-SHAH).—This expression is not, as is sometimes assumed, the contraction of *entre chaque temps* (to enter each time), but has been borrowed by the French from the Italian. In the old Italian School of Dancing, the raising of both feet, combined with the trembling battements (Italian, *battute*) of one foot or both without crossing, was called CAPRIOLA—CABRIOLE. We may mention that this form of battement is still in use in stage-dancing, and that the French School of Dancing, in respect of the execution of this movement, has adopted the technical term of *friser la cabriole.*

At a later date, the crossing of both feet (which was adopted about 1730 by the then renowned dancer CARMAGO) was called CAPRIOLA INTRECCIATA—*interwoven cabrioles,* and from that originates the word *entrechat.*

It is a brilliant dance-step, now reserved for theatrical dances, and always produces a fine effect. Formerly it was also executed in the ballroom, in the contredanses and gavottes. La Carmago doubled the effect of the step by executing five and seven entrechats terminated with an attitude. Later, in 1750, Mdlle. Lamy did seven and eight entrechats without effort. From 1766 to 1800 the step became so common that complaints were made to the theatrical managers about artistes employing them on any and every occasion.

Entrechats are divided into two sections—the even numbers 2, 4, 6, or 8, and the odd numbers 3, 5, 7. The former are terminated by alighting on both feet, the latter by allowing one foot to remain in the air after the spring. Entrechat in two (or á deux) is a simple changement de pieds (change of the feet) ; entrechat in four (or á quatre), in six, in eight, (á huit) the feet cut back and front two, three or four times during a single spring in the air. In the odd numbered entrechat—á trois, á cinq—the feet change three or five times, and the dancer alights on one foot, while the other is crossed in front or rear, or raised perpendicularly or horizontally to the supporting leg. It is indispensable to prepare for entrechats with a strongly accentuated bend of both knees before gathering sufficient force for the upward spring. Both legs co-operate in the movement of the entrechats.

Entrée (AHN-TRAY).—The opening of a dance ; the entry. Also a person's first entrance into society.

Entretaille (AHN-TR-TIE).—The jump preceding any step : jump on one foot, raising the other to the height of the waist. Old title, *entre la taille.*

Épaulement (AY-POLE-MAHN).—The shoulder. The movements of the body in opposition to the movements of the legs.

Epicredios.—Grecian country dance much in use among the Cretes, who danced it quickly, fully armed.

Epilenios.—Danced by the Greeks at country fêtes. Athenée and Pollux mention the dance. In the Pastorale of Longus the following description is given. " Dryas stood up and ordered a bachanalian air to be played. He executed the dance of the winepress, successfully imitating the vintagers carrying the back-baskets filled with grapes, then crushing the grapes, filling the barrels, and drinking the sweet wine. The movements of the dancer expressed all this with such reality that the spectators believed they saw the wine-press, the barrels, and that he really drank the wine."

Equerre, *en avant, en sautant* (jumping).—For Jigs, Hornpipes, etc. From the 3rd position, bend both knees (*plié*), in rising, spring forward on the soles, and open the heels outward, place the heels on the ground, turn on them, raising the toes a little, and open the toes outward. Repeat this en avant, then en arrière.

Equilibre (EKWI-LIBR).—The fundamental principal of perfect poise or stability, whether standing on both feet, or only one. It is the perfect balance of the whole body accomplished by regular, graceful carriage of the upper body, and preserved by its independence from the feet, yet working together in harmony.

Escargot.—*See* Farandole.

Espardageta.—Steps used by clever Catalanian dancers. It is a typical Spanish step, and consists of a very rapid battement of the heel against the instep. Notwithstanding the rapidity of the movement the action should be easy and graceful. The pas espardageta reminds one of the French little battements on the instep.

Été (AY-TAY).—The name of the second figure of the Quadrilles, and owes its origin to the steps executed. It was once the custom to make the figure with a step composed of a chassé, a jeté, an assemblé devant for the avant deux. The union of these three steps is known as *pas d'été.* The figure was for some considerable period known as the avant deux, because the two dancers—lady and vis-a-vis gentleman—advanced when commencing it. *See* Quadrilles.

F

Failli, *pas.*—A step executed as follows :—Make three quick small walking steps and finish with both knees bent and remaining in that attitude. It represents the movement of a person who risks falling to the ground. It is done en avant, en arrière and á côté.

Faler.—Dance 1879. Tempo, 2-4. *Position:*—Gentleman with r. holds lady's l. hand, both facing forward. The couple make five slow pas glissés, then the gentleman makes the lady do an allemande (8 bars). Repeat. Then 4 steps forward in pas sautés (4 bars), change hands; r. hands joined make a tour de main to right (4 bars). Four pas sautés (valse á deux temps sauté) (4 bars). Change hands, l. hands joined. Tour de main to left and four pas sautés. Release hands, both pirouette. Reverence, and recommence.

Fandango.—This may be considered a true type of Moorish and Spanish dance and a relic of the voluptuous dancers of antiquity. It produces a magical effect on the dancers and spectators in exciting their temperament. At the first accents of the music men and women become fascinated in a manner unknown in the West. The dance varies in different localities; the fandango of the ballroom also is different to the one danced on the stage where grace is displaced by free gestures which often give the dance a shameless character. It is usually danced by one couple to music in a quick 3-4 tempo accompanied by castagnettes. The noise of the castagnettes, the agitation of the arms and hips and tapping of the feet add to its originality and character of life and action.

Fandango for the Ballroom, for 4. 8, 12 or 16 couples. 126 bars of music in 3-8 time, with 5 bars introduction. Castagnettes in each hand are used to accompany the music. [PAS DU FAN-DANGO. Glide r.f. forward, draw l.f. up to r.f., glide r.f. forward; repeat commencing l.f. (2 bars).]

Introduction 5 bars. *First Figure*, 16 bars played four times (64 bars). Bars 1—16. All, playing with castagnettes without interruption, form two grand circles, gentlemen an outer and ladies an inner circle. Gentlemen move round to the right with pas du fandango and ladies round to left, On meeting partners they turn round each other and return to places.

Bars 17-32.—Ladies stand still while gentlemen with pas du fandango move backward to the centre of the circle finishing facing partners (4 bars). All fandango step to right, repeat to left, repeat to right, repeat to left (4 bars)). Take partner's right hand and fandango step round each other one way then the other (8 bars).

Bars 33-48—Ladies make a grand circle, with fandango step, outside the gentlemen and round to left (8 bars) and return to places. Gentlemen repeat round to right (8 bars).

Bars 49-64.—Gentlemen kneel on right knee. Ladies in centre back to back, then fandango round the gentlemen. Gentlemen rise and reverence.

Second Figure. 32 bars.—Gentlemen take ladies l. hands in their right and one pas de fandango to the left and one to the right, then the gentlemen make the ladies pass in front of them from the right to left for a change of partners, the gentlemen continue with the lady on the right two fandango steps and pass to next and so with all the ladies.

The ladies come back to their partners, who make them do one or several pirouettes in place, according to the steps of the dance and the number of couples taking part (this figure is arranged for eight couples only). If it is danced by 16 couples, the fandango step must be omitted, and only one is done to the right and then the pass. Play of castagnettes with one hand and grand salute.

Third Figure. 30 bars.—Each gentleman gives his r. hand to his partner's l., and describe a grand circle around the ballroom, the two fandango steps (2 bars), they stop and leave each other, play of castagnettes with both hands, knocking them together (with the castagnettes) after each bar (2 bars). Repeat these four bars to the end, then the gentleman makes his partner do a pirouette. Bow and curtsey (finale).

Fandango, *au Théatre.*—Tempo, 3-4. This dance is executed by the couples being placed opposite each other; they accompany themselves with castagnettes, making steps and gestures which depict all the passions. Thus it is a pantomime, in which the gentleman makes a declaration of love to the lady. She repulses him, he seeks to win her, she flies. He becomes furious and stamping his feet swears to win her at any price. She turns on him and mocks him; he in an extreme rage, renews his declaration. This time she accepts him, and after several gestures of love and content they execute the following *vis-a-vis.*

1. They describe a grand circle then change places by pas glissés, alternating on each foot.

2. They turn round each other, and return to their places by pas glissés chassés with the same foot.

3. Lift r.f. in 2nd elevation, ditto l.f. Repeat 8 times with attitudes and play of castagnettes; turn, with a bend of the body to one side, hands describing a circle. Repeat 4 times to each side.

4. Lift r.f. en avant in 4th position, assemblé, glisser l.f. 3 times en arrière, drawing r.f. up after each glissé. Repeat 4th part 4 times, taking it up from commencement and doing 2nd, 3rd and 4th. Gentleman puts one knee on the ground and the lady seats herself on the other.—Attitude to finish.

Farandole or **Farandoulé**, also known as **L'escargot.**—Originated in Provence, France, and flourished till the end of the eighteenth century. It is now rarely seen. The step was a galop step (glissé-chassé) and the figure was a chain formed by the dancers who were led by a conductor. All the dancers were linked in a long line and wound in and out like a snail (escargot) and then unwound, going round obstacles and even up and down stairs, practically, a "follow-the-leader."

Festius.—An ancient Greek family festival dance. Originally it was danced by the family itself, afterwards professional dancers were employed, the family joining in at the end of the repast.

All sang and danced together. Xenophon gives the following description of the Festius:—

"Directly the meal was carved the libations made, and the hymns sung, a Syracusan entered with a flute player beautiful and well-made, a dancer who executed perilous springs, and a youth who danced whilst playing perfectly on the lyre. The dancer advanced into the dining room to the sound of the flute. She was given twelve rings, and began to dance, and throwing them in the air with so much accuracy that as they fell back into her hand they marked the rhythm. A large circle was then brought in ornamented with daggers pointed inwards, into the middle of which the dancer executed a grand spring, which caused great astonishment and fear to the spectators who thought to see her perhaps wounded. But she executed this with her accustomed address and without doing herself any harm. The youth then danced his gestures and movements making him even more pleasing to the onlookers. A parasite seated at the feast got up trying to imitate the movements of the youth and the dancer, but in such a way that all his gestures appeared ridiculous. The dancer then made the wheel by turning her head towards her feet. The buffoon in imitation bends forwards and does the wheel in this position. The youth was covered with applause because he gave, in dancing, the whole action of his body. The buffoon demands a livelier tune from the flutist, and at the same time moves his feet, arms and head until thoroughly exhausted he fell on a couch."

Fêtes.—From the most primitive times we find traces of dancing in all the private, public, official and national fêtes and festivals. In Athens and Rome the number of dances were as great as the number of fêtes, and each had its special name and character. As to our fêtes, we know that dancing is their particular aim and ornament. Even in religious fêtes, the history of religion and its customs, we find the first essays on dancing, and the more one advances in the history of religion the more it is mixed with the dance. At Aix, on the occasion of the Fête Dieu, we find dancers mentioned. Chérunel in his interesting "Dictionary of the habits and customs of the people," divides the fêtes in which dancing takes an important part under five different heads. 1. Fêtes with a religious or popular character. 2. Knightly and warlike fêtes. 3. Fêtes exclusively for the populace. 4. Court fêtes. 5. National fêtes. We find the dance in all public, private, official and national rejoicing.

Large processions which we still see with banners, bands and songs, are only really reproductions of the moving (ambulatory) ballets of the middle ages. The word *procession* is derived from the Latin *procedere*, which means to march to time with rhythym and order in which one sees the idea of the dance, that is, order and regularity of movements. We still find in village churches reminiscences of these ancient ceremonies. We see the choir march past with slow steps in time to the music before the preacher commences the Credo. In the antique fête of the fire of Saint Jean dancing appears again when we hear of the villagers dancing round lighted wood fires, carrying away the burnt wood and preserving it till the next year as sacred to the fête of Saint Jean.

In the provinces of Ninervais and Bourbonnais the weeping bands which accompanied the funeral ceremonies are equally a tradition of dancing.

Feu, *danse du*—The fire dance is very prevalent amongst the savages of Oceania, who took such a pleasure in it that they continued during entire nights round immense braziers. A dancer holds a lighted torch to prove that the fire is still alight. Sometimes they dance carrying the brazier in their mouths. The Jesuit Pere de Charlevoix mentions this dance in his "Voyage en Amérique Septintrionale": "A Missilaqui regaled us with a singular fête, which had something rather pleasing about it; it was quite night when he entered into the hut of a savage with us. We found a lighted fire, near which a man beat, whilst singing, a kind of tambourine, another shook, without ceasing, a chichikoné, singing at the same time. It lasted two hours, which bored us extremely, because he always repeated the same things, that is to say, he formed half-articulated sounds which never varied. We prayed the master of the lodge not to 'continue this prelude further, and he had great trouble in telling us he would not. Then six women appeared, standing in a line side by side very stiffly with arms hanging. They sang and danced without disturbing the line, making a few steps to time, sometimes forward, sometimes backwards. This lasted a quarter of an hour, and the fire which alone lighted the cabin was put out, and nothing could be seen except a savage dancing with a lighted torch in his mouth. The music of the chi chikoné was not discontinued, and the women took up from time to time their songs and dancing. The savage danced all the time, but as he was only distinguishable by the lighted coal in his mouth he made a spectre horrible to behold. This mixture of dances, songs, instruments and fire which never went out, had something bizarre and savage about it which amused us for half-an-hour, after which we left, the hut, but the game lasted till daylight."

Figure.—This expresses alike for ballroom and theatrical dances the union of several steps and the changes, by one or several people. It is also the figure described on the floor. Dance figures are composed of several changes forming a homogeneous whole, as, 1st, 2nd or 3rd figure of the parts composing the entire dance.

Filette, *la.*—Name of an ancient contredanse used at balls before the quadrilles, we find the name only no details.

Finale.—The last figure of Quadrilles.

Flechir (FLAYSHEER).—To bend.

Fleuret (FLER-AY), *temps.*—A fencing foil. Name of an ancient dance-step often used in old contredanses and the old passe-pied. Diderot's encyclopædia gives this description:—" Fleuret is not like the bourré because it has only one movement. It is easy to execute and consists of a demi-coupé and two pas marchés on the points of the feet. It is done in the 4th position. If l.f. is forward the weight of the body is entirely on this foot drawing r.f. in the 1st position without its touching the ground. Then bend both knees equally (*plier*). You must not pass r.f. in front in 4th position until after the bend, and at the same time as it passes lift yourself up on the points. Afterwards two pas marchés on the points one with l.f. then r.f. on the last place heel on ground to finish it so that the body is firmer either to take another step or to do the first step again according to the requirements of the dance. The fleuret is also done en arrière, de côte, á droite or a gauche. It is only positions which differ.

Flexion.—The bending of any of the joints.

Flic Flac.—Starting with the r.f. in the 5th rear, bend the knees and pass it to the second elevated stretched, then with a jump throw it against the l.f. which is sent to the 2nd position on the ground, the weight of the body falling on the r.f.; this terminates the pas. This pas has but one temps and gliding the r.f. in the 5th front, we shall be ready to repeat it with the other leg. Bending the knees, the l.f. which is in the rear passes to the 2nd elevated poition, and, with a jump, is thrown against the right sending it to the 2nd position, the weight of the body falling on the l.f. and this terminates the pas. It is performed sideways to the left when starting with the r.f. and to the right when starting to the left.

Flore, *pas de.*—Known as *pas ordinaire.* From 1st position, (and) hop on l.f. simultaneously raising r.f. (1) Glide r.f. to 4th forward with dégagé (2) Hop on r.f. immediately carrying forward l.f. in preparation for the next step.

Flore, *danse de.*—This dance, originally graceful amongst the Greeks, fell to a point of the greatest obscenity amongst the Romans. Métius had it danced one day in the presence of Cato when the Roman courtesans refused to appear before so severe a censor. The people witnessed his discontent when Falconius, the friend of Cato, predicted it would meet with scant approval from spectators. Cato understood and escaped, not wishing to be a witness to the excesses of the Danse de Flore. Until its death floral games and scenes were established in their primitive splendour and grandeur.

Folatre, *la*—Name of a square dance, composed by the celebrated Blasis, master of the ballet. The authority of this clever master resulted in its being adopted in several salons. He leaves the following directions:—(1) Demi-chaîne anglaise. (2) balancé. (3) demi-chaîne anglaise. (4) balancé. (5) four gentlemen en avant. (6) four ladies en avant. (7) chassé-croisé les huit. (8) ladies chain. (9) chasse á quatre sur les cotés. (10) balancé. (11) tours de mains. (12) two couples return. (13) chassé en avant quatre. (14) return to your places repeating the chassé. (15) balancé by the eight. (16) tours des deux mains. (17) the same for the other six. (18) altogether, repeat. The Folatre was danced by four couples and the music was played four times.

Folies d'Espagne, *les.*—Dances in Spain, are executed by one person alone as a sarabande. The folies d'espagne were danced to the sound of the castagnettes and the flute; the dance, quick and light composed of quick steps, show the meaning of its name. Feuillet in his "Choréographie" gives the music and the theory of the Folies d'espagne for one woman alone. It is written in 3-4 time and contains principally the blacks and the crochets to facilitate the movements of the feet rapid and staccato. Later on the name Folies d'espagne was given to a contredanse in 1830, when it had some success. As we do not see it figure in any quadrille of the epoch, it must have formed a complete dance and not a figure introduced into a contredanse or quadrille.

Forez, *danse de.*—An ancient French proverb, deriving its name from the dance. Compan in 1313 says, Guy, Count de Forez, after having met Philip le Bel at the great assembly held by that king at the fête at Whitsun, returned home to Forez followed by a large number of his suite. On his arrival he gave a grand fête, with which dancing was connected. The flooring gave way and many of the guests were hurt. Some even did not survive their injuries, hence comes the saying "Danse de Forez" to express a great joy followed by a great sorrow.

Forlane.—A dance very much danced in Venice by the Gondoliers. It is also called the Foulane; it is very animated and danced to a 3-4 time. The forlane draws its name from

Fione, the land of its birth. It very much resembles the tarantella in which there are little close steps and glissades coupés.

Fouetté, *temps* (FOO-ETT AY).—Whipping time. Name of a very brilliant dance-step, especially beautiful when executed by dancers whose legs are well turned out. Stand in 5th position r.f. in front; bend the knees, jump on l.f. at same time lifting right leg de coté horizontally outstretched; bend the left leg a second time while the r.f. crosses in front or at the back of the left leg, according to whether the fouetté is done in front or rear. Note that this step is done on the 3rd beat of the polka mazurka.

Fourchette, *pas de la* (FOORSHET).—Fork l..f is raised forward with an imitation of a tap of a fork in the r. hand which is formed by the index and middle fingers being apart while the other three are closed. The body is tilted forward, l.f. raised forward and tap with r. hand, then backward.

Frangesa.—Dance by R. M. Crompton, composed to music of this name.

Frapper, *pas frappé* (FRAHP-PAY).—To beat; a beating step. If, when taking a step the floor is stamped. It can be done with any part of the foot. It is also known as *taper* a *tapé*.

Frappé tortillé, *pas* (FRAHP-PAY TOR-TEE-YAY).—Tortillé is to wriggle or twist. (1) stamp r.f. in 2nd position with dégagé. (2) l.f. turned inward on the heel before the other foot. (3) turn the foot outward. These two turns of the foot are tortillé; combined with the first (beating step) it is the frappé tortillé. *See* Tortillé.

Frotter, *temps* (FROTTAY).—To rub. Rubbing one foot against the other or any part of the leg during a step.

Frou-Frou Mazurka.—The lady, at the right of her partner, leans her l. arm on his r. shoulder, he places his r. arm round her waist.

(1) 8 *bars.*—The gentleman and lady do two pas de mazurka with l.f. en avant (2 bars). Take up the position of a couple dancing and execute an entire turn by two pas de redowa (2 bars). Repeat these two pas de mazurka and the rotation (4 bars).

(2) 8 *bars.*—The gentleman taking lady's l. hand in his left, and her r. hand in his right do two pas de mazurka to the left (2 bars); they release l. hands and do two pas de redowa taking up the position usual in that dance (2 bars). Then, the lady turns round the gentleman passing beneath his arm (4 bars). If it is an entire turn with the l. hand the gentleman simulates a pas de boston sur place, while the lady turns round him.

Funambules.—Name given by the Romans to tight rope walkers dancing on the rope, the Greeks often replaced this word by that of acrobat.

Funeral Dances.—These go back to the greatest antiquity. Though in modern times we should be very surprised to find such a dance forming part of such ceremonies, they formerly played an important part. Plato tells us that in the obsequies of the kings of Athens, a troup of chosen people arrayed in white vestments opened the march. Two rows of young men walked in front of the coffin and two rows of virgins. All wore crowns and branches of cypress; they executed grave and majestic dances to lugubrious tunes. The musicians walked between the two groups, and behind walked the priests and different divinities. Among the half-savage people of Canada funeral dances still play a great part, and commence the moment the body is enclosed in the piece of wood which serves as a coffin.

G.

Gagliarde, *pas de* (GAHL-YARD).—This dance-step commences with either foot in the 3rd, 4th or 5th position and terminates in the 2nd position. It consists of an assemblé in the 1st position followed by a step to 2nd position.

Gaillarde or **Galliard,** known also as **Romanesca.**—A dance that came westward to Paris and London in the sixteenth century from the Roman Campagna, where it is still in favour. It was also known as *cinque pace,* or five steps, and one remembers that Beatrice, in *Much Ado About Nothing,* refers to it when she speaks of courtship as "hasty, like a Scotch jig, and full as fantastical"; the wedding as "a measure full of state and ancientry"; and subsequent "repentance," who "falls into the *cinque pace* faster and faster till he *sink* into his grave." The dance was lively to music in 3-4 time, the dancers singing love ditties. Two couples were placed *vis-a-vis* as in the French quadrilles, the gentleman taking the lady's hand. Promenade with pas marché springing, and lifting the shoulders gaily; assemblé with each foot, then glissade, jeté and assemblé. These steps are done en avant, en arrière, to right, to left, in crossing to change places; bow and curtsey after each part and conclude with a promenade. As the Romanesque or Romanesca it was danced leaping in the air and lowering to the ground, crossing gliding or springing. The steps were quick, varied and infinite. Each dancer exhibited his talent and ardour in springs, cabrioles, wheels, glissés terre-à-terre, small sautés, pas marchés, tombés and assemblés, Arbeau (1588) devotes a long chapter to this dance. Diderot's "Encyclopædia" gives this description—"The step is done en avant, en arrière and de côté; to do it en avant stand with l.f. in forward 4th position with the weight of the body on the heel of r.f.; levé; from this bend on l. leg raised, lift yourself to spring. Then cross in front in 3rd position coming down from the spring on both feet, knees straight; the foot which was crossed in front is carried to 4th rear with the weight on it raising yourself at the same time."

Another description. (1). (Not hand in hand, but separated). Spring from one foot to the other, with the raised foot in elevated 5th position, four times. Echappé to the right in turning (2 bars). Repeat four times, echappé twice to right, then twice to left (16 bars altogether).

(2). *Pas de bourrée* three times to right, three times to left, three times to right and three times to left. Dancers cross each other.

(3). *Coupé dessous* (pas de bourrée). Coupé dessous with r.f. (2 bars) r.f. pas bourrée (2 bars) pas bourrée l.f. (2 bars) pas bourrée r.f. (2 bars).

(4). *Coupé dessous, pivoter.* Coupé four times (2 bars), pivot to right four times (2 bars). Repeat twice.

(5). *Temps levé, tourné.* Cross r.f. over l.f. Rise on toes and turn slightly to left. Repeat with l.f. over r.f. Repeat eight times. Each figure is of 16 bars of music.

Galop.—Dance more ancient than is generally supposed, dating back to the end of XVIII century. It served as a finale to the voltas and contredanses, a character which it still maintains. After the slow and reposed movements of the older dances, the dancers rejoiced in more animated movements assisted by faster and agitated music, thus accelerating the dance. The word " galop " expresses the fastest running of a horse; the word " galopade " formerly expressed the dance, but in later times " galop " has been more usual, " galopade " being understood to mean simple sideway chassés and " galop " the waltz-like twining with chassés alternately. The music is 2-4 tempo. The step is of the most simple nature and consists of a glissade (glide) with one foot which is chasséd with the other so as to continue without changing the foot. To turn in the galop, alternative chassés must be made, turning a half-circle on each second beat thus:—*gentleman's step* (1) glide l.f. to left (*and*) chassé l.f. with r.f. (2) glide l.f. to left pivoting a half-circle on it (1 bar) repeat with other foot (1 bar); *lady's step*, the same with the other foot.

Galopade Russe differs from the Galop in never being danced in turning. The dancers galop rapidly round the room making their partners advance and retire only with either simple or alternative chassés to music in 6-8 tempo.

Gauche (*à gauche*) (AH-GOHSH).—To the left.

Gavotte (GAH-VOT).—Originally a peasant dance from Gap in Dauphiny, where the natives are called Gavots. At the end of the fifteenth century the French Court commenced to dance it in costume. The oldest description extant is in the " Orchesography " by Thoinot Arbeau (1588). The music is said to have been composed by King Louis XIII of France (1601). The " classic " gavotte, however, was composed by Gaetano Vestris and is known as " Gavotte de Vestris," at the beginning and end of which there is usually danced the introduction of " Menuet de la Reine " arranged by Gardel (1770) to music by Rameau. It was danced by a single couple, the gentleman commencing by presenting the lady with a bouquet followed by a kiss; this custom is, however, ignored by such writers as Noverre and Cahusac. In the figures, the dancers exhibited their choregraphic talent in the most varied and fashionable steps of the period such as, pas de basques, jetés, bourrées, pas de zephires, entrechats, brisés and glissades, endeavouring to be particularly brilliant in the solos.

Gavotte.—To the music " Le Ballet du Roi " by Lulli (1633-1687). In common time commencing on the 3rd beat of the bar. For one couple. (1) Four gavotte steps forward, four gavotte steps round, four gavotte steps back and four round again, the dancers holding the inside hands and turning the head and body toward and away from each other in accord with the step. (2) Gavotte round the room, the lady changing place four times with deep bows and curtsies. (3) Facing each other, take both hands and alternate toe and heel step; point toe in front, then rear, then up the room, pivot, same back and pivot. (4) Repeat same step to the right twice, twice to left and four gavottes round. (5). (1) Glide one foot forward (2) glide the other foot to rear (3) point the first foot to side (4) point the same foot in 5th position. Repeat this movement four times and four gavotte steps round each other. (6) Gavotte step forward three times, pirouette and repeat. The *Gavotte step* is made by taking (1) a gliding step forward (2) close the other foot to 3rd rear (3) glide first foot forward again (4) raise second foot to 4th front.

Gavotte de Vestris.—Introduction—the first part of " Menuet de la Reine." (*First figure*—8 bars). Temps levé to 4th *forward,* assemblé dessus l.f. changement de jambe sauté (2 bars) 3 jetés dessous *backward* and assemblé dessus (2 bars). Repeat the 4 bars making 8 bars in all.

(*Second figure*—8 bars). Crossing each other, gentleman to rear of lady, 3 glissades croissés dessous, dessus, dessous (2 bars). Backward 4 ailes de pigeon (2 bars). Repeat same 4 bars re-crossing.

(*Third figure*—12 bars). In place, the following step is made with a half-turn to the right to the lady. Balloté dessus et dessous, pas de zéphire; repeat the step with the other foot, repeat again with l.f. and again with r.f. (8 bars) 4 jetés dessous (2 bars) assemblé, entrechat, entrechat (2 bars).

(*Fourth figure*). Repeat last 12 bars commencing with the other foot, but making the last four bars to move away from each other to the left finishing at the opposite left hand diagonal corners of a square. These four figures constitute the first part of 40 bars. The second part consisting of 40 bars is composed of the Solos for the dancers, as follows: —

(*First figure*). Solo for the Gentleman, 8 bars. R. pas de basque forward, L. pas de basque forward (2 bars). 3 pas bourrée and assemblé backward (2 bars). 2 pas de basque forward (2 bars) 2 pas de basque pirouette backward (2 bars).

(*Second figure*). Solo for the Lady, 8 bars. Same as gentleman's solo.

(*Third figure*—12 bars). Gentleman commence r.f. lady l.f. Balloté and zéphire thrice (6 bars). Balloté and assemblé with gentleman making a quarter-turn to left to finish opposite to lady (2 bars). 4 glissades croisés to the left (2 bars). 2 jetés dessous and assemble (2 bars).

(*Fourth figure*—12 bars). Repeat third figure. Following this is the third part also of 40 bars.

(*First figure*—8 bars). Temps levé sauté forward, contretemps dessus, changement de jambe (2 bars) 4 temps de cuisse alternately (2 bars). Repeat 4 bars.

(*Second figure*—8 bars). Cross, gentleman passing rear of lady with chassé, pirouette (2 bars). 4 ailes de pigeon (2 bars). Repeat re-crossing (4 bars).

(*Third figure*—12 bars). Ronde croisé, gentleman to right, lady to left, with pas balloté and two temps fouetté, repeated three times (6 bars). Balloté and assemblé in place (2 bars). Backward 4 jetés, assemblé and 2 changements (4 bars).

(*Fourth figure*—12 bars). Gentleman to left with ronde croisé step of 3rd figure but commencing l.f. (6 bars). Balloté and assemblé dessous with r.f. in place (2 bars). Moving back to original places—4 ailes de pigeon, assemblé, 3 entrechats. Then repeat the first part of " Menuet de la Reine " to finish.

Gavotte de Stephanie, *pas de.*—Common time, commencing step 1 on the introductory note (fourth beat).

(1) Glisser r.f. obliquely to right en avant.

(2)   „   l.f.   „   „   „

(3)   „   r.f.   „   „   „

(4) Bring point of l.f. to point of r.f. bending the knee. Repeat with other foot. This step can be done in every direction and turning.

Gavotte-Quadrille, Gavotte Kaiserin, or **Gavotte l'Imperatrice.** Berlin 1893. Obtained remarkable success in Germany. Recalls to the spectator all the graceful moods of the menuet. Executed by four couples as in a quadrille to music in common time by P. Hertel. Révérences, balances, pointes, pirouettes and enchaînements of hands are its principal features.

Explanation of the steps. PAS BALLOTÉ :—From 1st position (1) raise r.f., knee outward, point of toe turned down and must not touch the floor and close to l. ankle, glisser r.f. to 4th front. (2) degager (free) the l.f. and bring it back to 1st position and raise it. (3) glisser l.f. to 4th front. (4) repeat temps (2) of this bar. BALANCÉ DE LA GAVOTTE (1) from 1st position glide one foot to 2nd position (2.3) the tip of the other foot glides to 4th forward at same time turn forward the side of the body corresponding to the foot. (4) Pause. PAS DE BOUTS. From 1st position. Two of these are done to one bar of music. (1) glisser r.f. to 2nd position head and eyes directed to the point of the foot. (2) close l.f. to r.f. (3.4) Repeat with other foot. PAS GLISSÉ.—From 1st position. Glisser point of a foot to 2nd position. (2) close the other to 1st position. (3.4) repeat with other foot. PIROUETTE.—From 1st position. (2) place one foot forward to 4th position. (2) cross the other foot over in front (3) pivot on the soles in the direction of the first foot (4) lower the heels.

THE DANCE. Introduction—révérences (4 bars). The couples now place themselves in a square. The gentlemen conduct their ladies to the centre face to face by two pas ballotés. The 1st step is begun with the r. foot. The 2nd step is begun with the 1. foot. (3) Two pas ballotés begun with the r. foot. Lady and gentleman change places, l. shoulder to l. shoulder. (4) two pas ballotés. Begin with r. foot to return to place. (5) one balancé to the right. Join l. hands. (6) one balancé to the left by the r. hand.. (7) two pas ballotés begun with the r. foot. A half-turn with r. hand is executed. (8.9.10) repeat (5.6.7). (11) four pas ballotés begun with the r. foot. By these four pas ballotés is executed a turn of the two hands. At the end the gentlemen go to the centre and give the l. hand to opposite gentleman. The 4 couples thus form a star (or moulinet). (12) two pas de bouts with the r. foot and with the left. (13) the couples, beginning with the r. foot, make, by 4 pas marchés, half-turn en avant (in a star). (14—19)—Nos. (12.13) are repeated three times. (20) two pas ballotés with the r. foot and finish in the 1st position. (21) two pas ballotés, begun with the r. foot, lady and gentleman giving each other r. hand, next to each other, go en avant and presenting the opposite couple who are coming towards them, the gentleman his l. hand to the lady without letting go of his lady's hand. By this is formed the Rosette. (22) pas balancé to the right. (23) pas balancé to the left. During these two steps the opposite couples look at each other beneath the raised arms to the height of the face. (24) two pas ballotés, begun with the r. foot, ladies and gentlemen dance en arriere, and the ladies present to the gentlemen vis-a-vis (opposite) who are coming towards them, the l. hand without releasing their right. (25) pas balancé to the right. (26) pas balancé to the left. At the 4th temps lady and gentleman turn themselves suddenly one towards the other (vis-a-vis). During these two steps the couples look at each other beneath the raised arms to the height of the face. (27) two pas glissés á gauche (to the left). (28) pirouette begun on the l. foot. (29) two pas glissés to the right, the smallest possible, so that the lady and gentleman find themselves nearly vis-a-vis. (30) pirouette begun with the r. foot. (31) the gentleman stretches, during the 1st and 2nd temps, his r. hand to· his lady, who during the 3rd and 4th temps, stretches her r. hand to him. (32) the lady executes with the l. foot a pirouette; the gentleman with the heels slightly raised makes his partner turn. (33) release hands and execute a révérence de gavotte to the right. (34—37) Nos. (21—24) are repeated. (38) the couples in front separate from those at the back, and beginning with the r. foot they execute two pas ballotés going towards the couples to the side. Those at the side in the same way execute two pas ballotés. All the dancers turn themselves en avant, and at the end they find themselves vis-a-vis (face to face) on two lines per couple. (39) 4 pas ballotés. The dancers execute a traversé (they change places). (40) retraverser (in the same way. (41) 2 pas ballotés. The ladies go the centre and form a " moulinet " (by the r. hand): the gentlemen going next to them so that lady and gentleman are l. shoulder to l. shoulder. (42) a quarter-turn of " moulinet," the gentlemen moving to the right the ladies to the left by 2 pas ballotés. (43) a turn of the l. hand with the lady *vis-a-vis* by two pas ballotés. (44—49) The Nos. (42—43) are repeated three times. (50) révérence to the lady, gentleman conducts by " pas marchés " his lady to the position of the first figure. Révérence. The gentleman takes back his lady and they separate.

Ghost Dance.—This dance was the main cause of the Indian rising in the North West, when the famous Sitting Bull lost his life.

Gigue.—*See* Anglaise. 2-4 tempo—16 bars for each step. For 1, 4, 8, or 16. (1) promenade to right (*See* Matelotte). (2) pointé, ciseaux (scissors). (3) berceau, eight times en avant and en arrière. (4) pointé en tournant to right and to left. (5) three battements with the sole of r.f., berceau; repeat with l.f. (6) tombé and three changements de pieds. (7) scissors turning to right and left. (8) sissones in turning and glissades to right and left. (9) tombé, piqué and assemblé to right and to left. (10) battements of the sole, berceau of r.f. and repeat with l.f. (11) jump en avant, scissors, three changes of the heels and repeat en arrière. (12) stretching of r.f. berceau en avant; repeat with l.f. (13) échappé, entrechat, ciseaux with r.f., assemblé changment of the heel; repeat with l.f. (14) berceau in turning to the right and to left. (15) ailes de pigeon in front, berceau; repeat to left. (16) ailes de pigeon coupé forward with r.f., ditto l.f.; repeat. (17) ailes de pigeon in place. (18) écart, entrechat, tour en l'air, entrechat and attitude.

Glissades, Glissés. These stepe are used both in stage and ballroom movements. The foot can glide in any direction. By the term *pas glissé* is understood a step sideways and a gliding of the other foot. Temps glissé is made by raising on both feet, fall back on one foot and glide the other in any direction.

Glissade soutenue.—The foot glissé is raised before the other in 3rd position instead of remaining on the ground at the end of the glissade.

Glissé, *temps.*—This temps is made by gliding forward or backward quickly drawing the other foot to it. *Glisser* is the verb to glide, glissé is a glided step.

Grace.—The ideal of the pure and highest beauty of movement which can appear in the human body and the wonderful attraction which captivates every eye. Grace is a beauty which is not given by nature, but is produced by the subject; the beauty of the human form honours the creator of nature, grace its owner. The former is a gift, the latter a personal merit founded on the inner harmony of æsthetic conditions and the full expression of living movement. Grace makes itself apparent through its endeavour to please naturally, lightly and without effort. To exceed the free measure of nature produces affectation. Dancing provides the means for the acquirement of grace, giving the body ease in its waving and undulating movements. Slow and long-drawn movements are, of course, best for this object. "The dance-teacher assists real grace in giving to one's will the power to subjugate the body, and in removing the obstacles with which matter and weight obstruct the play of living forces. He can do this only in accordance with rules which keep the body in healthy limits and which as long as laziness opposes will appear stiff and forced. But when the teacher dismisses the pupil the rule must have done service so that it need not accompany him into the world, in short, the working of the rule should have entered his nature." (Schiller). This fascinating human ornament may be a production of art if it is not a gift of nature.

Graces, *les.*—A dance in the early part of the nineteenth century, since obsolete. A gentleman placed between two ladies gives his hands to right and left; the ladies joining left and right hands in front. The three advance and retire several times, then salute. The gentleman makes the right lady pass under his r. arm; he then makes the same " passe " with the lady on the left; the three form a circle and terminate in retiring, the gentleman being placed between the two ladies. The dance is derived from l'Allemande.

Grand (GRAHN).—Large; meaning to fullest extent. The word is usually prefixed to a step or movement which it is intended should be performed to its utmost limit. Thus " grand rond " grand circle, that is all dancers join hands in a circle; " grand rond de jambe," the largest circle it is possible to make with the leg, etc.

Grave, *pas*; or **Pas de Courante.**—*See* Courante. This pas at one time was called de COURANTE on account of its being the principal pas of a remarkable dance called by that name and which was performed at the magnificent Courtballs, but it lost that name and began then to be called pas GRAVE; later, the MINUET having its origin among the peasants of the French Province of Anjou, came into great vogue under Louis XIV. and superseded the COURANTE, which fell entirely into disuse.

The Pas grave may begin with either one or the other foot in all five positions and usually terminates, travelling forward, in the fourth, and sideways, on one side or the other, in the second, and returning from the second into the fifth position. It consists of three movements; the first is a plié, the second the rising and the third the sliding gently with the toes on the ground. It is the equivalent of one bar of music the accent of which falls on the second movement. To execute the pas grave forward from the fourth to the same position with the r.f., place the weight of the body on the l.f. holding the right behind on the toes, bend the knees raising at the same time somewhat the r.f. from the ground meeting the l. heel with the instep in the third position; then raise again the r.f. in the air in the second position describing a small circle and finally slide forward with the toes into the fourth position. If you wish to make this pas forward from the third to the fourth position starting with the r.f. in front of the left, it would be necessary to bend, rise, and glide in a straight line into the fourth position. The same pas can also be made sideways, but not backward in ballroom dancing. En tournant, do not exceed a quarter of a circle.

Gromenard.—The name of the Japanese salute, which is much deeper than the reverence of the West. It is made by bending the upper part of the body so low that the brow nearly touches the ground.

Group.—The placing together of several persons according to their height, direction, appearance and colour so that they constitute a harmonious whole or unit.

Grue (GRU).—A crane, bird. Jump on l.f., raising r.f. to 4th forward, cross it in front of l.f. This can be done with both feet and in all directions.

Grue, *danse de la.*—An ancient dance of the Greeks. often mistaken for " la candiote;" it was held in the open fields in the first days of Spring. Boys and girls danced various figures, approaching and receeding one to another, forming rondos. The dance concluded by a kind of farandole conducted by a couple holding each other with a ribbon under which every dancer passed. Every one then rolled themselves around the couple and the lady of this couple raised the ribbon as a sign of release; on being unrolled every couple took to flight. The dance of the " grue " represented the labyrinth (maze) of Crete, and must have been invented by Theseus. It is known that Theseus, after having deliverd the Athenians from the domination of the Cretans, halted at Delos, and after a sacrifice offered to Venus danced with the young Athenians this dance of the " grue." Callimaque in his hymn to Delos mentions this dance of the " grue " attributing its creation to Theseus, and leads us to believe that it was thus called because it recalled a flock of cranes flying behind each other, dispersing and uniting again before continuing their flight.

Guarachas.—Dance in Spain, and executed to the sound of a guitar. from which its name is derived. From the quickness of its steps and the character of its poses it seems to be derived from the Moorish dances.

Guerre, *danse de.*—War dance. This war dance is described by Cook in his travels, and he states it to be scattered among the less civilized tribes of South America. The dancers form a ring and the spectators sit round them. The dance being started by one man is continued alternately by all the others. This dancer seems to spring to the right or to the left, while singing some war exploit; his gestures are military and full of energy; with a club he then knocks vigorously a post placed in the centre of the ring and is accompanied by musicians striking cymbals. This dance is enacted principally before war expeditions to inflame the tribes with courage.

Guimbarde.—Compan's dictionary gives this name to an ancient dance; owing to the lack of information we are only able to mention its name. (Guimbarde also means in French an old worn out cart or carriage). This is, perhaps, why bad carriages in Paris are named thus, because they jolt and bump the passengers, recalling a disorganised dance.

H.

Haiva or **Heiva.**—Dance of the Tahitians, in which gentlemen and ladies take part one after the other. The ladies shine with their grace and the richness of their costumes; their abundance of hair in long plaited tresses which are artistically arranged on their heads, the arms and the neck being bare; the breast is decorated with shells or bunches of feathers and their body covered with a white dress trimmed with brilliant coloured borders. The movements of the Haiva are slow, measured and precise; arms and legs vigorously observe the measure of the tom-tom and flutes. These dances more often take place in houses addicted to this pleasure; a large roof, supported by beams of wood, surrounded by a palisade decorated with tapestries elevates itself over a large hall covered with matting on which sit the spectators, the centre being reserved for the dance. In the centre stands the " patan " or master of the ballet, who indicates the different figures of the dance which are often continued very late in the night.

Hare.— Dance of Siberia, in which the natives pretend to be hares and imitate the frolics of those animals.

Harrovian Waltz.—By R. M. Crompton.

Hea.—Oceanic dance, well known among the islanders. Is fairly difficult, being composed of numerous gestures and accompanied with original songs. The choir consists of ten or twelve chiefs in a circle in the centre of which is another who, with a pair of sticks, beats the time on a plank about ten feet long. This time-beater makes the dance go fast or slow as the whim seizes him but always ending with very rapid beats when the dance is simply a mad frolic. The men dance round the choir with simple stamping steps, pausing now and again to assume some graceful pose. The natives consider it imperative for the chiefs to dance this well as a mark of good breeding and which lends an air of dignity to the dancer.

Heartsease.—A formal, tender, old English dance for two couples in a circle. They meet with four steps forward then backward, 8 bars. Repeat. The men retire from their partners, meet again and turn once round, 8 bars. Retire again and advancing turn partners with l. hands, 8 bars. Form line with partners and the opposite lady. Repeat 4 bars—8 bars. Take arms with partners, turn, then turn the other lady, Repeat, 8 bars.

Hedion.—Ancient Greek lascivious dance accompanied by song.

Hermes —A pantomimic dance, consecrated to Mercury, and representing the actions of that god.

Hermites.—Branle. Dance of the middle ages, classified among the high or jumped dances. The participators formed themselves into a single file and followed the movements of the leader.

Highland Schottische.—Round dance for one couple; 2-4 time usually the music is based on Scotch airs. The dance is divided into two parts of eight bars each. The dancers face each other and with the l. hand over the head and the r. hand on the hips the first part is performed thus: (1) spring r.f. to 2nd point, (2) r.f. to 5th rear, (3) r.f. to 2nd point, (4) r.f. to 5th rear, (these four steps are accompanied by a hop on the l.f.) (5) glide r.f. to 2nd dégagé, (6) l.f. to 5th rear, (7) r.f. to 2nd dégagé, (8) hop on r.f. Repeat the whole reversed; 8 bars in all. The second part—lock r. arms and with l. hands over the head do the following going round (1) step on r.f. (2) hop on r.f. (3) step on l.f. (4) hop on l.f. (5) step on r.f. (6) hop on r.f. (7) step on l.f. (8) hop on l.f.; now change arms and hop four the other way. Repeat *ad lib.*

Hilaria.—Dance festival in honour of the god Pan, which took place in calends of April.

Hilarodes.—Dancers whose costumes consisted of a long white tunic; on their heads they bore golden wreaths and on their feet a simple sole held on by strings.

Hiporchromatic dances, so called on account of their rhythm, their figures and movements. They included all the Lyric dances as well as the accompanying songs which were consecrated to Apollo, as well as the so-called Dithyrambic dances.

Histrions.—Derived from the Tuscan word "hister," signifies the dancing actors who came to Rome to inaugurate the scenic games. They sang simple verses or recited them accompanying the words with suitable dance movements or gestures. More often two histrions appeared and while one recited the other danced.

Hit or Miss.—Old English dance for eight in two lines. All advance and retire, repeat. Then all advance again with a double, that is, four steps forward and back closing the feet to the left *vis-a-vis* partners changing hands and then meeting again, taking their own partner's hands and into their places, all four doing Grand chain. Then the two sides advance and retire and repeat. Each take the other's arms and repeat as before.

Holubiec.—*See* Czarine. Dance-movement employed in the Mazurka to signify "the turn on the spot" preceding or terminating a figure. After or before each figure the gentleman passes his r. arm round the lady's waist and turns with her on the spot; he quickly changes his arm by passing the lady in front of him. The step is made in three temps (1) raise r.f. to 2nd and let it down to 3rd rear (2) pause with knees bent (3) again raise r.f. and stretch out both legs. Lady does the same with opposite foot. Russians often dance the holubiec holding the lady's hands crossed behind her back instead of holding at the waist, the direction is also changed by releasing hands to change sides and retaking the hands.

Hongroise (HON-GRU-AHS). Hungarian national dance, introduced about 1800 as a complement to the Gavotte. The natives always dance it in their spurred Hungarian boots, their spurs, however, carrying only round molettes (rowels) without spikes to avoid injury to the lady's dress. The steps are the same for gentleman as for the lady. Two ballonés in front or side and three small temps currus on the tips slightly jumped. Figures of the Hongroise: —

Promenade: The gentleman leads his partner by the r. hand and promenade *ad lib* round the room. *La Valse*: He takes the lady by both hands, facing her, and turn together with the Hungarian step with alternate feet. *Le Balancé*: Releasing hands they make the step facing each other advancing and retiring in place. *La Poursuite*: He advances towards the lady while she retires round the room; after a few times he retires while she advances always with the same step. *Valse Finale*: They join hands crossed in front of them and turn together as if waltzing. The music is 2-4 tempo, strongly accented, even a little jerky, and is so appropriate and Hungarian in character that the dance could not be danced to any other music.

Hop.—*See* Sauté.

Hoplomachie.—Greek pyrrhic dance with shields.

Horai.—Greek dance, symbolising the seasons. According to Xenophon, at the commencement of the autumn, the Grecian youth, crowned themselves with purple and ivy, formed processions taking abrupt steps and accompanied by the sound of fifes and drums, the gestures and chants expressing the greatest mirth. At the return of Spring, they adorned themselves with crowns of oak and roses, the women being lightly dressed and adorned with flowers, danced pastoral dances. They simulated the innocence of the early times by simple and modest steps. At harvest time, new festivals recalled a happy and abundant harvest. When winter came this dance united the families in their homes.

Hormos.—Greek dance, combining the greatest dignity and most rigid behaviour.

Hornpipe.—This is certainly an English national dance, although associated with sailors and called the "Sailors Hornpipe." But there are many hornpipes and hornpipe tunes both in common and triple time with a special stress on the final note. It owes its name to the music which was played on a pipe with horn rims. The steps are as follow:—(1) first round (2) double shuffles (3) toe and heel (4) echappés (5) rocks (6) dips (7) slide toe and heel (8) scissors (9) hauling boats (10) rowing (11) climbing ropes (12) running rocks (13) running on the heels (14) last round, etc.

Houras.—Dance of the natives of Haouai in Oceania, representing scenic games with pantomimes.

Hydrophories.—Greek sacred dances danced to the "festivals of the deluge."

Hymen, dance of.—Greek matrimonial feast dance.

Hypogees.—Egyptian paintings recording family dances are thus called. All of them together with hieroglyphics are useful in the history of ancient dances. In some of them may be seen a dancing-master surrounded by equilibrists, dancers and gymnasts.

Hypogepones.—Greek tragic dance, depicting old people, bent with the weight of their years, leaning on sticks.

Hyporcheme.—Greek tragic dance, military according to some writers, of slow and stately movements.

I

Iambic.—The priests of the god Mars danced this in his honour, style slow and grave.

Igdis.—Ancient authors were unanimous in condemning this Greek comic dance, in which the dancer indecently agitated the hips.

Imperial Quadrille.—Enjoyed some popularity for several seasons, but on the death of the Prince Imperial of France its popularity waned and the dance is now obsolete. It consisted of five figures for eight people in the form of a square as in ordinary square dances. (*Figure* 1)—La Nouvelle Trenitz. (*Figure* 2)—La chaine continue des dames. (*Figure* 3)—La Corbeille. (*Figure* 4)—La Double Pastourelle. (*Figure* 5)—Le Tourbillon.

Inconnue, known also as "**l'Inconnue à la redoute,**" was danced as a quadrille towards the end of the eighteenth century.

Innocence, *danse de l'.*—Grecian religious dance, instituted by Lycurgus in honour of Diana and executed by young girls dancing round that goddess' altar.

Ionian Dance.—A slow, soft, effeminate, and sometimes voluptuous dance of the Ionians. It also formed a part of the sacred dances of the greeks. Originally the Sicilians practised it in honour of Diana, and Horace mentions it in his verses:—

> Motus doceri gaudet ionicos
> Matura virgo.

Italic.—The principal *Pantomime* dance of the Romans, and created by Bathylle a freed slave who improved on a dance of the Tuscans. He associated himself with Pylades, a clever actor whom he met in his travels in Asia Minor and at their joint expense they 'built a theatre for the production of Pantomime. Borrowing from various dances they invented the "Italic" and with the assistance of music represented tragedies, comedies and satires. Bathylle excelled in the tragic and Pylades in the comic line. They both enjoyed immense popularity although their rivalries often divided the capital of the Roman empire and they were often exiled.

Ithyphalles.—The ancient Grecian dancers who represented drunken men. They were clothed in a white tunic with violet sleeves

84

and over the tunic a very fine woolen drapery descending as far as the heels. They sang drinking songs while jumping about.

Ivrogne, *pas de* (IVRON).—A step forward or sideward on the heel.

J

Jaleo de Jarez.—A Spanish dance of the bolero type, with castagnets, by a man and woman. In rapid 3-4 or 6-8 tempo. Like all Spanish dances indolence and easy grace are its principal characteristics.

Jalouse.—An old French quadrille, danced for some time towards the end of the 18th and beginning of the 19th centuries. It was composed by Blasis.

Jamaica—Old English dance from Playford's " The Dancing Master " (1651). Standing in two lines lengthwise, the first man takes his partner by the r. hand then with l. hand and so change places. He repeats this with the two ladies and the first lady does the same with the two gentlemen and falls back into line so that the first couple are in the second place. Then perform the figure 8 to the end of the line. The first man then repeats it all commencing with second lady and so all down the line.

Jarreté.—*See* Bow-legs.

Javelote.—Military dance of the Greeks, so called because it was danced with " javelots " (javelins) and simulated the movements of attack and defence. It was practised by men alone.

Jeter, Jeté (ZHETTAY).—The outward spring performed by the throwing of one foot in one of the open positions and alighting on the same foot in a single beat. It may be executed in all directions as well as in place. Preparation—5th position r.f. in front. The l.f. is raised and thrown sideways to 2nd position while r.f. remains suspended in the air in the rear of l.f. Made to the side it is called " jeté ouvert." *Theory of three jetés assemblés. First jete*—raise the r. leg stretched en avant, slightly to the right. Throw the r.f. forward on the ground, and raise l.f. to the rear parallel with the r. leg. *Second jeté*—repeat the same movements with the other leg. *Third jeté*—same as the first. *Assemblé*—the l.f. is placed in front 3rd position during a light hop on the r.f., both feet flat. These jetés can also be made en arrière by throwing the foot backward, also to the side and turning.

Jeté, *petits battements.*—Jeté r.f. en avant, then bring back l.f., touching r.f. in rear, then in front of the r. shinbone (tibia) during one beat.

Jeté Attitude.—When the jeté is accompanied by any pose in which the body remains motionless; the dancer must become immobile immediately the jeté is terminated.

Jetés Battus.—The opposite leg to the one making the jeté beats against the other front and back during the jeté. On the stage this movement produces a most brilliant effect, particularly if the agility and suppleness of the dancer are such, that the whole length of the body can be placed horizontally during the spring. Example:—Stand in 3rd position, then in a single beat, spring as high as possible throw the r. leg forward on the ground and during this throw beat the l.f. against the r.f. front and rear as often as possible. Experienced dancers can beat three times before the tombé (fall). The movement somewhat resembles an entrechat, but the spring is done on one leg only, whereas in the entrechat the spring is on both feet.

Jeté étendu.—Beginning with the r. leg in a well-stretched forward 4th position, spring throwing the r.f. on the ground simultaneously throwing l. leg to 4th forward elevation; then throw the l. leg on the ground raising r. leg forward and continue progressing forward.

Jetés, *grands.*—Are made like small jetés, but the legs are more stretched, the elevations in the air are higher and the jump more distant.

Jetés, *grands developpés.*—The raised leg is developed horizontally to the height of the hip and then thrown forward or to the side. It is often used to prepare an attitude, an arabesque or a pirouette.

Jeté en tournant.—Bend l. knee with r. leg in 2nd elevation : throw the r. f. to the floor simultaneously turning half-circle to the right and raise l.f. at rear of the right. Do the same with the other foot.

Jeté Moucheté.—Make a jete, and before making another, with the other leg make a moucheté, front, or rear, or both.

Jeté Passé —From 5th position : bend the l. leg, and stretch the r. to 4th elevation forward, and throw it (jeté) in the 4th position on the floor, while the l.f. passes rapidly to 4th forward elevation. It can be made in all directions.

Jeté Tourné.—The leg making the jeté is placed, in turning, to the right or left, pivoting on one's self ; this jeté is often taken as the first temps of a grande pirouette, giving the necessary spring for the force of the movement required for the action of rotation, when the body can turn on itself several consecutive times.

Jéte Grand, *associated with a* COUPÉ.—The *jeté forward* is prepared and preceded by a coupé dessous; the *jeté backward* by a coupé dessus.

Jeu de la baguette.—Greek step. Each dancer grasps a stick, which is placed handy for the occasion. The first dancer advances with a long jeté of the r.f. and strikes the stick of the dancer on the right who strikes the dancer on his right and so on for all the others, then all the dancers make a jeté en arrière to return to places. Then they make some " pas de basques " with the sticks held over the head.

Jig.—The name is commonly derived from *giga*, or *gigue*, by which early fiddles were known. Early specimens of the dance

are found in " My Ladye Nevill's Virginal Book," dated
1591. The typical rhythm was dotted crotchet, quaver,
crotchet; the form was usually written in 3-8, 6-8, 3-8, or
12-8, and consisted of two repeated sections of four or eight
bars each. The dance attained its greatest favour with
musicians in the Stuart period. It became the closing movement of sets of dances, concluded stage performances, and
was used usually when sailors left their native land. With
the advent of Handel the English form declined. It would
appear that the jig went to Scotland and Ireland from
England. The dance known as " The Port " in Ireland preceded the jig in Ireland, but the rhythm of this differed from
the English jig. " Whatever the Irish jig was, it was certainly not called jig until the seventeenth century." The English
jig was introduced to France by English musicians who
studied there, and was used fitfully by Lully and much by
Marais. When the form reached Italy it lost its character-
istic rhythm and acquired the triplet figure, in which way it
was much used by Vitali and Corelli. In Germany the jig
was cultivated from the middle of the seventeenth century
onward. It was treated with great freedom by Bach, who
made it an integral part of the suite. The dance is very
exhilarating, the foot striking six or more times to the bar.
To clearly describe each step is almost an impossibility.

Jig, Kemp's.—This jig derives its name from Kemp, who was a
celebrated actor, describing himself as one who spends " his
life in mad jigges." It starts in a circle of six. During
two phrases of music, one man leads forward two ladies and
back. He bows to each then turns the third. He leads his
own partner with l. hand and the lady he had turned; repeat
with the other two ladies and turn his own partner. This
is done by the next man, then by the third man. For the
second part the first man again leads the ladies as before,
turns half round with both hands and repeats with own
partner; repeat with each lady; each gentleman repeats the
whole. For the *third* part the first man takes lady as before
crossing hands behind lead lady forward and back, turns
half round and throws her a kiss, repeat with next lady, turns
the third; each gentleman repeats.

Jig, Solomon's, or Green Goose Fair.—Old country dance for
eight dancers who stand longways. Advance and retire with
what was known as " single step "—two steps and close both
feet. Then, form two sides and turn with a single step.
Take each other's arms and turn single step. First couple
cast off, *i.e.*, turn down to right and left, meet at end of
line and pass up it back to their places, last couple repeat.
First couple go down between the lines and return on the
outside, last couple repeat. First couple with the single step
do the Hey—similar to the modern Grand Chain—on their
own sides, the others remain in their places. Each couple
repeats. In Chaucer's time (1340—1400) the movement of
the Hey was known as " the Reye " and was danced in a
circle, it is possible that it formed a complete dance.

Julie.—An old obsolete French quadrille.

K

Kalabis —Sacred public dance of the Spartans in the temple of Diana songs of the same name accompanied the gestures of the dancers.

Kalabrismes.—Greek warlike dance, with javelins and armour.

Kalenda or **Calenda.**—Danced by the Spaniards of S. America. The postures and gestures are lascivious in the extreme. Father Abbot in his travels gives the dance a religious character, affirming that the nuns practise the dance in the churches in the middle of the processions and during the Christmas offices.

Kaleustes.—War dance of the Greeks.

Kallikas.—Name of a step or perilous dance of a lascivious character, danced by Grecian women at private feasts and family festivities.

Kallimak.—Grecian dance in honour of Hercules.

Kalumet.—Dance in vogue among the North American Indian tribes, the Othagos and the Sakis; it is of a military type as all these tribal dances are. Warriors only are admitted, their bodies are painted with the most varied colours and heads adorned with feathers.

Kanake.—Grecian theatrical dance.

Kangaroo Dance of the aboriginal Australian, in which the chase of the kangaroo is accurately depicted in dumb show from the start to the finish.

Kapria.—Grecian military dance with shield and javelin.

Karyatis.—The invention of this dance is attributed to Pollux.

Kastachok.—Russian national dance in Ukraine. The dancers make noisy and precipitate steps sometimes accompanied by folly and intoxication. As in mazurkas, the heels are knocked together marking the tempo with a sharp noise, the dance being a symbol of vigour and energy.

Kateris.—Lucien mentions this as one of the earliest Grecian dances, and consists simply of gestures of the arms and hands.

Kemp's Jig.—*See* Jig.

Kermaphoros.—Grecian dance in which the dancers appeared to be in a fury; the name is derived from a kind of vessel carried by the performers.

Kideris.—Dance of the Arcadians at family festivals.

Kallinic.—A pantomime dance of the Greeks. Represented the descent of Hercules to Hades.

Klopeia.—Greek dance, little known.

King Edward's Lancers.—By R. M. Crompton.

Knismos.—Classed by Athene among the Grecian private dances, executed to the sound of the flute.

Knossia.—Dedalus was, it is said, the inventor of this dance. Young people of both sexes join hands and sing hymns in memory ot the victory of Theseus over the monster Minotaur.

Kola.—War dance, deriving its name from the dancers holding naked swords in their hands.

Kolatiskos was a procession of adults carrying baskets, and keeping strict time with the rhythm of a chant.

Kolo.—Austrian dance, a description of which is given in " Figaro " of February, 1883. This ascribes the dance as a native of Bosnia and that it became a craze in Vienna and as popular as the czardas. There is much of stamping and knocking the heels together. It is danced to the sound of the " guzla."

Komatik.—Grecian village feast dance.

Komos.—Grecian pastoral dance.

Konisalos.—Grecian comic dance.

Korabanthia.—Dance of the Corybantes.

Krakoviak, Cracovienne.—*See* Cracovienne.

Kreon Apokope.—Grecian dance, in which butchers cutting up meat were imitated.

Krinon.—Grecian dance of the choirs in the tragedies.

Kronsthiron.—Grecian satirical dance of the theatre.

Kybele.—Grecian satirical dance, representing Cybele in the arms of a shepherd.

Kybistesis—Cretan dance with the heads bent low.

L

Labalette.—Ancient obsolete French Quadrille, consisting of chassé made en avant and turning, executed by four couples.

Laconien.—Grecian dance in vogue among the Laconians from which it derives its name. It was composed of three choirs who sang and danced a representation of the past, present and future.

Ladies' Chain or Chaine des Dames.—*See* Quadrilles.

Lancers, or **Les Lanciers** is a Quadrille of English origin. The invention is ascribed by some to Joseph Hart and others to a publisher named Duval of Dublin. It was introduced about eighteen years after the French Quadrille. It consists of five figures bearing fanciful French names without any particular meaning, as follows:—No. 1, *La Rose*; No. 2, *La Ladoiska*;

No. 3, *La Dorset*; No. 4, *L'Etoile* (more generally called " visiting "); No. 5, *Les Lanciers*.

The name and forming of lines in the 2nd figure would suggest that the inventor intended to give their movement the character of a Polish dance; while the joining of hands, curtseying, etc., in the 3rd figure savours of a good old English country dance. The culmination of the dance is of course in the last figure from which the whole dance takes its name: here it is to be urged, that the gentlemen when falling in lines, crossing behind the ladies and re-crossing and wheeling to the left in Indian file should be most precise and soldier-like in their movements, instead of shuffling in a bored and aimless manner through what can be made a really pleasing sight to spectators.

Lancers (Duval's).—*The original descriptions are here given.*—

1st. First lady and opposite gentleman chassez to the right and left and swing quite round with r. hand to places—les tiroirs—the gentlemen join l. hands in the centre and r. hands to partners and ballotez—change places with partners, ladies join r. and l. hands in the centre, ladies dance round to the left, and gentlemen go round outside to right—turn partners to places.

2nd. First couple advance twice, second time leave the lady opposite—chassez right and left and turn partner—right and left, balancez to sides—advance in two lines and turn partners.

3rd. First lady chassez forward and stop, then opposite gentleman, both retire en Pirouette, ladies hands across gentlemen's going round with partners.

4th. First couple with lady on left advance twice—set and pass between the two ladies, hands three round and back to places.

5th. Grand chaine—first couple turn half-round with their backs to the opposite couple, the side couples follow in turn, forming two lines—chassez croisé all eight and back—ladies lead round to right, gentlemen to the left, meet partners and lead up the centre—set in two lines, gentlemen on one side, ladies on the other, turn partners to places—the grand square.

Lancers, Hart's.—

1st. Opposite lady and gentleman advance and set—turn with both hands, retiring to places—top couple lead between the opposite couple—return leading outside—set and turn at the corners.

2nd. First couple advance twice, leaving lady in the centre, set to partner in the centre—turn partners to places—all advance in two lines—all turn partners to places.

3rd. First lady advance and stop, then the opposite gentleman—both retire turning round—the ladies hands across quite round, at the same time the gentlemen lead round outside to the right, all resume partners and places.

4th. First couple set to couple at their right—set to couple at their left—change places with partners and set back again to places—right and left with opposite couple.

5th. Chain figure of eight half-round, the same repeated to places, the first couple advance and turn facing the top, then couple at the right advance behind top couple, then the couple at the left and the opposite couple do the same, forming two lines, all change places with partners—back again—the ladies cast off to their right, while the gentlemen cast off to their left—meet and lead your partners up the centre—set in two lines, the ladies in one line and gentlemen in the other—turn partners to places—(*all promenade at the finish*).

Lapithes.—A dance of monsters, half men, half horses.

Lascives.—In favour with the Greeks and Romans both in public and private life. These dances, which were innumerable, were most licentious in their nature.

Leda.—Classified by the Greeks among the dramatic and tragic dances and represented Jupiter changed into a swan. In spite of its severe character, the dancers assumed indolent attitudes.

L'envers.—Reverse, as *valse à l'envers*, reverse waltz. Sometimes termed à rebours.

Levé (LEV-AY) Raised, as applied to the stepping leg. The leg may be raised either en avant, en arrière or à coté.

Levé, temps.—A raising time. Raising one leg with some movement of the other leg.

Levé Sauté.—A jump, falling on one foot while the other remains raised.

Lever (LEV-AY).—The lifting of a leg, the opposite is *baisser*, lowering· (*See* Abaissements).

L'été (LAY-TAY).—The second figure of the Quadrille. Either single été or double été, occupying 24 bars of music.

Lionne.—Terrible and tragic dance of the Greeks.

Longue, la.—Dance dated 1760. Tempo 2-4. All the dancers in a long row, join hands. Then crossing one foot over the other they glide eight steps to the right and repeat to left. All the men advance to form a front line, then both lines change places, then go en avant to form a single line and farandole, and repeat the whole *ad lib*.

Louis XV (Danse de), 1725. by Louis XV.— 16 bars of ¾. The gentleman, with his right hand takes the left hand of his lady.

1*st.* The gentleman begins with the l.f. and the lady with the right, they execute four pas glissés en avant (4 bars).

2*nd.* The gentleman releases the lady's arm and offers his l. hand to her l. hand, and make a turn together with four pas glissés (4 bars).

3*rd.* The gentleman offers his r. hand to his lady's r. hand, and makes her execute an allemande making her pass under his r. arm (4 bars).

4*th.* The gentleman with his r. arm entwines the lady's waist, and execute the waltz sauté (4 bars). Repeat *ad lib*.

Louŕe.—A kind of ronde with slow movements. The name is derived from the instrument used to accompany it, somewhat resembling a bag-pipe.

Ludions.—Greek singing dancers from Etruria.

Lysiodes.—Greek women dancers dressed in men's clothes. The dance was devoted to the worship of Bacchus.

M

Macabre. dance.—So named after its inventor Macaber, but it is asserted authoratively that the word is derived from "make or break." The dance had a certain amount of success and was a public representation of persons of both sexes under the emblem of death. In its movements the character was both philosophical and moral. Its mimicry attempted to prove that equality unites all in the grave. In 1422 the "danse macabre" was performed before Charles VI. of France and Henry IV. of England and their Courts. The dance was printed for the first time in 1486 entitled "La Grand Danse Macabrée des hommes et des femmes" (the great dance Macabre of men and women). The painters Durer, Holbein and Gorgon have traced on canvas the tragic and allegorical movements of the dance.

Mackter and **Macktrismos.**—Grecian lascivious and licentious dance.

Maestoso.—Majestic—either dance or music, as Gavotte, Menuet.

Magnesien.—Grecian rustic dance.

Magodes.—Grecian dancing men in women's clothes. Their songs and dances were passionate and lascivious.

Mahony, quarré de.—Old XVIII century French Quadrille Eight dancers advance together and retire. Four went to sides and again retire. The sides then advance to first and second couples while the first four chassé-croisé to right and left. The first four execute some chassés-ouvert to the side, all being the same side, while the second four advance, etc., and repeat.

Maitre de **ballet.**—Ballet-master. He must combine the choreographer (writer of dances) librettist (writer of the plot) musician and artist. The famous masters of ballet were Blasis, Noverre, Gardel, Dauberval. Two distinguished ballet masters were Saint-Léon and Petitpas in whom the science of the ballet was inborn and whose work recalled the mïse-en-scène (staging) of the great Italian Masters.

Among the Romans the ballet master had need of all the treasures of intelligence and soul because he lacked the resources of decorations and stage properties to which we are accustomed. The enlightened taste of Roman art was very difficult to satisfy in stage dancing, and this gave rise to many dissensions and discussions. Lucien initiates us into the attributes of the ballet master, " he should be acquainted with poetry, music, geometry and philosophy."

Manchegas.—Quick, gay, Spanish Dance in demand by the general populace, and seldom seen in the ballroom.

Marché, pas (MARSHAY).—A marching or walking step; known also as *pas allé*. This step can be either half or whole. The half-step when the foot goes forward from the 1st position to the 4th, the whole step when it goes from the 4th rear to the 4th forward.

Marriage dances are used by every savage tribe in S. America. The newly married couple dance in front of the guests at the wedding repast.

Masquerades.—Dances or other functions in which the participators wear masks. The word is derived from " Mascarade," buffoonery.

Masques.—The ancient spectacular shows from which the modern ballet originated. They consisted of dialogues, songs and dances. The dresses were not always correct but the speeches were very brilliant. The first trace of " the masque " is dated Henry II. (1100) for Christmas celebrations. Henry VIII., Elizabeth, James I., Charles I. and II. patronised the masques.

Masur, Masurek.—*See* Mazurka.

Matassins, dance.—Dance practised by jesters in the middle ages The movements were very varied but unskilful.

Matelotte (sailor) Promenade.—From the Gigue and Anglaise. 8 bars 6-8 tempo. The dancer crosses the arms in front of him or places the hands on the hips. Others grasp the end of a stick (with both hands) over the head and during the dance lower one end under the r. arm, the tip behind the back, the l. hand being then free is placed on the hip.

The dance. Bend on l.f., stretch r.f. en avant to 4th position. Hop on l.f. and place point of r.f. to toe of l.f. Hop again on l.f. slightly developing r.f. in the air, then quickly bring point of r.f. to toe of l.f. Spring on r.f. by throwing it en avant and stretch l.f. to 4th avant. (1 bar). All this has been done during one bar, that is the two hops and the two small battements in front followed quickly by the " jeté developpé." Repeat it with l.f. Repeat all three times, that is four times with each leg alternately.

Continue the dance with " Berceau " Trot de Cheval, Corde, Ciseaux equerre (square) by jumping en avant and en arrière, écart on the heels (tramping on the heels), berceau turning, pirouette and final attitude.

Matelotte des Mousses of the cabin boy. Cabin Boy's Hornpipe· Tempo 6-8. Generally by one person, but any number may take part.

1st Step. Promenade de Matelotte (see last article), then jeté en avant r.f., jeté en arrière l.f., three changements of the heels, two chassés ouvert, contretemps to the left, pirouette to left, demi-face and pirouette to left, pas de corde, (attitude).

2nd Step. Two chassés ouvert, two temps zephyr, pirouette to left, pirouette to right, two temps zephyr, tombé three times, pirouette to left and écart trépigné.

3rd Step. Four temps zephyr, two chassés ouverts, contretemps to left, pirouette to left, contretemps to right, two temps zephyr, contretemps, two temps zephyr and demi-face. (Demi-face is made in a quarter-circle making a contretemps and a pirouette to the left).

4th Step. Four temps zephyr, four grands battements to right and left, two chassés ouverts; two temps zephyr, pirouette to left and to right; two temps zephyr, pirouette to left, two temps zephyr, tombé three times, pirouette to left, pas d'ivrogne.

5th Step. Four temps zephyr, two chassés ouverts, contretemps to left, pirouette to left, contretemps to right, two temps zephyr, contretemps to left, two temps zephyr twice terre á terre.

Maxixe Bresilienne.—The Maxixe is composed of five figures which are easily joined together in the order indicated. But as in the Tango this dance is not phrased, and each dancer may at will join together the figures in a different order.

Position of the Boston.—The gentleman commences " en avant " with the r.f. and the lady " en arrière " with the left.

The lady executes the same steps with the opposite foot, except in certain " enchaînements " which will be described.

Introduction: The gentleman executes pas marchés en avant at the rate of one step per bar.

Example: *1st temps.*—Place the r.f. en avant the r. leg stretched out, the body slightly bent towards the right, the waist bent.

2nd temps.—Place the l.f. " en avant " leg stretched out, body bent towards the left.

Four or six " pas marché " are generally executed, and without stopping the 1st figure is attacked.

1st Figure: *1st temps.*—Place the tip of the r.f. " en avant " a little to the right, cross the l.f. behind the right and strongly bend on the l. leg. (This crossed movement is at the same time a " movement tombé ").

2nd temps.—Place the r.f. " en avant " a little to the right and at the same time straighten up slightly. Repeat the same movements starting with the l.f., etc. This figure is made while turning, that is to say in describing a circle, it lasts about 8 or 10 bars. (Be sure to accentuate the bending of the body at the movement of the " croisé-tombé "). This figure can also be danced by placing the heel first instead of the tip.

The continuation of the 1st *Figure*: " The chassés de côté." Having terminated the first part of the figure to the left, place the r. heel on the side, the bust inclined towards the same side, and bring back the left behind the right (1 temps). Repeat this movement three times with the same position of the body, then begin again these 4 temps with the l.f. by changing the position of the body, that is to say body inclined to the left. As already said, this dance is not regulated, and each step may be repeated for a more or less length of time, providing that the measure is kept. Generally, this figure is made once more before attacking the second.

Enchaînement.—In order to pass to the 2nd figure this " enchaînement " is the simplest and the most used. During the 4 chassés with the left the lady re-bends her r. arm and gives her r. hand to her partner's r. hand behind her waist, and both their l. hands join together over their heads, the arms slightly curved. In this position they still continue 4 chassés during which the dancer makes his lady turn slowly, in order that she will find herself placed, at the 4th temps, in front of him a little to the right. The gentleman will not make the 4th chassé, but bending slightly to the right he will pass his arm under that of the lady's who will lean on this arm and against the gentleman's shoulder. Left hand to l. hand, arms stretched out and to the shoulders height, r. hand to r. hand, the gentleman's arm under that of the lady who bends hers in order to lean and to give the hand to her partner. The body slightly bent en arrière. In this position they begin the 2nd figure. Both start off with the l.f. " en avant."

2nd Figure: 1st *temps.*—Place the l. heel " en avant," let the foot fall down again flat, weight of the body to the left, cross the r.f. behind the left far enough and bend strongly on the r. leg (the r.f. on the tip). (As in the 1st figure, the " movement croisé " is at the same time a " movement tombé ")

2nd temps.—Place the left to the left a little " en avant " in straightening up (the weight of the body to the left). Repeat these movements starting off with the r.f., etc. This figure may continue as long as the 1st.

In the course of the figure the dancer will pass from left to right of his lady and *vice-versa* in changing the position of the arms, but without any change to the steps.

Enchaînement.—In changing sides the gentleman will bring back his arm on the lady's shoulder, without releasing her hand, and placing himself a little more exactly behind her, he will continue the step, but much less accented, that is to say, almost without bending and by leaning to the right and to the left according to the movements of the feet, the eyes fixed on the face of his partner. She making the same step as his will turn slightly the head to the right and to the left while looking towards him. This part of the figure may be made to last 4, 6 or 8 bars, and on the last one which must be on the l.f., the gentleman lifting the arms will make his lady execute a half-a-turn who will find herself facing him. The lady must take this half-turn without changing her step and must find herself ready to start off with the r.f. The gentleman does not turn but is in readiness to commence with the left, having made the last bar with " pas chassés " with the left.

3rd Figure.—Face to face, the hands united and the arms lifted slightly curved, they will make four chassés going towards the left (for the gentleman). These " chassés " are identical with those of the 1st figure, but without bending the body. The gentleman will continue to make again four chassés, during which the lady will make a complete turn while advancing in the same direction as her partner and without releasing his hands. To execute this turn she will make a " pas de polka " on starting with the l.f. and then will make 2 " chassés " with the right to terminate at the same time as the gentleman.

Then they will repeat the first part of the 1st figure for several bars, then will begin again these chassés and this turn in the opposite direction. Begin once again the first part of the 1st figure, then the " chassés " towards the left in describing a circle and slowly lower the arms to the height of the shoulders but stretched out lateraly, then again make the first part of the 1st figure.

4th Figure.—This has some similarity to the Medio Corte of the Tango Argentin. It contains 2 measures or 4 temps. For the gentleman:—

1st temps.—Place the r.f. " en avant " and flat.

2nd temps.—" Glisser " the l. tip " en avant " and very slightly towards the right in turning the body a little to the right and " chassé " the left with the right.

3rd temps.—Place the l.f. " en arrière " in bending on the l. leg.

4th temps.—Rise on the tip of the l.f., lifting the r.f. a little from the ground. The lady executes the contrary movements, that is to say by starting with the l.f. " en arrière," etc. (She must not jump, unless it is a number for theatre or music hall).

To join this figure with the preceding one, 4 or 8 " pas chassés " are generally made.

To pass to the last figure the first part of the 1st figure is repeated.

5th Figure.—For the gentleman. Being in the starting position, after having made the first part of the 1st figure he places his l. heel " en avant " and brings nearer his r.f. towards the left (1 temps), then place the tip of the l.f. " en arrière " and bring closer the right, always continuing to advance towards the left.

The lady makes the same movements with the r.f., but to the contrary, that is to say tip " en arrière " while the gentleman places the heel " en avant." Then begin again the first part of the 1st figure and terminate with the 4th.

This is in brief the theory with the enchaînements. I hope my readers will be able to understand this dance which, without being difficult, requires a good deal of attention. Several teachers have attempted to describe it, but did not succeed in making anything tangible or authentic.

Advice.—Do not exaggerate the movements. Do not stretch out the arms too straight and do not lean " en avant " in the 2nd figure. Keep the arms slightly curved and well elevated over the head and do not go too far away from your lady to make her turn in the 3rd figure.

Maypole Dance. —From "Ancient Dances Revived." The Maypole was set up in pretty well every village in the good old times, the lads and lasses dancing round it. It took a prominent place in the May-day celebrations, and the Morris dances were greatly aided thereby. The peasantry went into the woods for the flowers wherewith to decorate the huge pole of extreme height which took a yoke of many oxen to draw it. They danced and they sang and made merry to their hearts content in all the country side, and even in Cornhill, where the may-pole was higher than the adjacent Church spires, and the dance was always hilarious, joyous and full of action, the streamers from the high pole floating in the breeze as the dancers in a circle, hand-in-hand, twisting in and out plaited and un-plaited the ribbons that hung from the top.   .   .   .

The block to hold the pole must be heavily weighted and have a revolving pivot at the top. About a dozen dancers is a suitable number, twelve men and women, each holding a ribbon suspended from the top which they carry as the maypole is brought in with much ceremony and sunk in the block.

Then the dancers dart away from the pole to the full extent of their ribbons, and manipulation of these streamers should be well studied beforehand, for if they become wrongly inter-twisted the whole effect is spoilt and it would be neces-sary to take the pole out of the socket or they would not un-plait.

Form a circle round the maypole, and measure ribbons from the pole in a straight line.

1.—Dance round without plaiting and reverse all round; do this twice; *throughout the dance all the movements are repeated reversed.*

2.—Dance a chain about the pole, plaiting the ribbons the while round in and out, and reverse to unplait. If not rightly done, the pole must be taken out before proceeding which spoils the effect.

3.—Ladies take their places and dance round the gentle-men who run to the centre and kneel on one knee.

Then the ladies trip to the centre and do the same, the gentlemen dancing round. This is followed by a pause of a few seconds the music playing the while, then everybody return to places with ribbons untwisted. All dance round in a plain circle without plaiting and reverse.

4.—Ladies to centre, ribbons outstretched held in both hands in front. All revolve round the pole, ladies back to back, reverse, and return to places. Gentlemen do the same. Then ensues about ten seconds pause, and the dancers measure their ribbons before they repeat the plaiting chain and reverse. Then half-minute's rest.

5.—Ladies trip to the centre taking hold of the pole with left hand and hold on firmly; gentlemen do same with right hand. Then reverse quickly and change hands afterwards. Forming a circle they go round without plaiting and reverse. Then all stop short, measure the ribbons, and put the ring attached to the end of all the streamers in the mouth, and holding hands, all go round very steadily and smoothly in a circle and reverse.

This is followed by a slight pause, the music continuing, then the men and women form a final tableau, and after half-a-minute's pause, trip away carrying the maypole with them.

Mazourka.—A Polish national dance performed by at least four couples or sometimes more in a circle, and is composed of numerous figures, the same as the Cotillon.

Mazurka Polka or **Mazur** or **Mazurek.**—So named from the Polish tribe of Masures in the former duchy of Masovia. Mazurka, translated into English, means Masovian woman. This dance is preferred, in the Polish countries, to all other dances. It is also danced in other countries in Europe. In England it has ceased to be a ballroom dance but still figures prominently in stage dancing. (See Holubieck.). It is composed of two parts of three beats each, occupying two bars 3—4 tempo. The first three temps are called " pas de mazurka " the second three temps are " pas de polka." A half-turn is made with everv two bars, that is, six steps, the turn being made on the second three steps. Assuming a count of six to complete the step, stand in waltz position:—

> For the gentleman
> (1) Glide l.f. to left.
> (2) Close r.f. to l.f.
> (3) Hop on r.f. and bring l.f. up behind r. heel.
> (2 and 3 would constitute a *chassé-fouetté* or *coupé dessous.*
> (4) Make the first step of the polka with l.f. ⎫
> (5)   "   second   "   "   r.f. ⎬ turning
> (6)   "   third   "   "   l.f. ⎭ ½-circle.

For the lady the same movements with the opposite foot. Now continue, the gentleman commencing with r.f., the lady with l.f. (4, 5, 6, will constitute the Redowa step).

Medopïsmos.—Ancient Greek tragic dance mentioned by Athene as being widely spread throughout Laconia.

Memphitique.—Ancient Grecian martial dance in armour, said to be invented by Minerva (mythology). As in the " Pyrrhic," the dancer arrayed with sword, javelin and shield executed all the movements of attack and defence, thus training himself for the military profession. The dance was divided into " gymnopedie " for the children and "enoplienne" for adults. They resembled the open-air drill of the modern schools, and were composed of two camps according to the dancers' ages. Martial poetry which accompanied the dance excited the dancer in " throwing the javelin " or shielding himself. Ancient authors divided the dance into—(1), The Podisme, a quick movement of the feet. (2), Xephisme, an imitation of a warrior either striking or shielding. (3), Leaps and bounds representing jumping over a ditch, hillock or rampart. (4), Tetracone, forming a square followed by marches and counter-marches.

Menuet.—(MAIN-WAY).—Often mis-spelled "*minuet.*" A dignified dance of French origin of the former Province of Poitou, for two persons executed on the figure of the letter Z, originally on the letter S. The name is derived from the French word *menu*, Latin *minutus* which means small or pretty, signifying the steps should be small and pretty. The music which, in 3-4 time, M.M. 54, should be very majestic with the accent well marked on the first and third beats. The music of most menuets is composed of two parts of 8 bars each, and a so-called trio of two parts of 8 bars each, as each part is repeated there will be altogether 64 bars, as the whole is played twice, the complete dance will be 144 bars. Many celebrated musicians wrote Menuets and that by Mozart from the opera " Don Juan " is famous. The order of this dance was first introduced by Pécour, a celebrated dancer (1674-1729) at the French Court, hence the name " Menuet de la Cour " ("Menuet of the Court "). The most beautiful of all the Menuets was arranged by Gardel for the wedding festivities of Louis XVI. and Marie Antoinette, which was therefore called " Menuet de la Reine " (" Menuet of the Queen "), music by Rameau. It was generally danced in combination with " Gavotte de Vestris."

Although it is no longer a ballroom dance and is even scoffed at by persons too ignorant to be able to estimate its worth, it is, nevertheless, considered an indispensable means of training by all really educated dancers and teachers of dancing, and reappears periodically in the drawing rooms of good society, which has yet sense and taste for the really beautiful. Again and again efforts are made to do honor to this queen of dances and wherever seen it is always enthusiastically received.

There are four composite steps which are peculiar to the dance:—

    (*a*) PAS DE MENUET À DROITE. Menuet step to the right.
    (*b*) PAS DE MENUET À GAUCHE. Menuet step to the left.
    (*c*) PAS DE MENUET EN AVANT. Menuet step forward.
    (*d*) BALANCÉ DE MENUET.

For purposes of instruction it is better to use two bars of music for each step, and count six.

    (*a*). MENUET STEP TO THE RIGHT. (1).—Glide r.f. to 2nd toe position. (2).—Dégagé, through which l.f. will become 2nd point. (3).—Bend (plié) r. leg, while l.f. glides to 5th rear. (4).—Dégagé to l.f. (5).—R. f. to 2nd position with dégagé. (6).—L.f. to 5th rear with dégagé. Two such movements usually follow each other.

    (*b*). MENUET STEP TO THE LEFT. *First Part.* (1) — Glide forward r.f. to 4th position with dégagé. (2).—Rise slightly on r.f. and simultaneously glide l.f. to 1st toe position. (3).—Lower r.f. and glide l.f. to 2nd point position. (4) — Dégagé, through which r.f. will become 2nd point. (5) — R.F. glides backward into 5th position with dégagé. (6).— Glide l.f. to 2nd position with dégagé. *Second Part.* (1).—

R.f. glides backward to 4th position with dégagé. This will restore the distance between the dancers. (2).—L.f. glides backward to 1st position. (3, 4, 5, 6,) same as in the first part.

(*c*). MENUET STEP FORWARD or en passant (*ahn passahng*(Preparation, as at end of last step, *i.e.*, 2nd position. *First Part.* (1).—Advance r.f. from 2nd position passing lightly near the 1st position into the 4th position with dégagé. (2).—Glide l.f. passing lightly to 3rd rear and into 2nd point position in the air (*en l'air*). (3).—L.f. glides forward into 4th position dégagé. (4).—Pause. (5).—Glide r.f. into 4th forward position. (6).—Glide l.f. to 1st position, dégagé. *Second Part.* The r.f. commences from 1st position and 1, 2, 3, 4, of the first part are repeated. (5).—R.F. is placed before l.f. in a well-crossed 5th position rise and make a half-turn to left. (6).—Lower the feet into 5th left forward position and withdraw it so that the r.f. is ready to move to the right. This half-turn causes the change of front.

(*b*). MENUET BALANCÉ. Preparation r.f. in 2nd position (1).—Pass r.f. into 1st and into rear 4th position dégagé. (2).—L.f. glides into 3rd rear. (3).—The same foot goes into 2nd elevation. (4).—Put down and glide l.f. passing 1st position into 4th rear, dégagé. (5).—R.f. glides backward into forward 3rd position. (6).—And glides and is raised into 2nd elevation.

In its complexity the Menuet indicates the three following principal movements. (1).—The Introduction. (2).—The dancing of the figure Z. (3).—Finale.

The INTRODUCTION is preceded by two révérences, one to the audience and one to partners. The FINALE is followed by two more révérences. It is a bold undertaking to give an exhaustive description of this dance as it would fail owing to the impossibility to describe its peculiar subtleties and the varied shades of its component blended parts. Notwithstanding this we venture on the following outline for one couple, assuming that the four principal steps already described are thoroughly understood and practised.

PRELUDE of MUSIC. 8 *bars*. Each gentleman leads his lady by the left hand to the selected place for commencing, stands at her left side and releases her hand.

1 *bar*. Both put r.f. in 2nd position revolving on it, and prepare for a révérence by lady drawing l.f. to 3rd front, gentleman to 3rd rear. At the first step of this, gentleman's r. hand takes lady's l. hand.

1 *bar*. BOW. (1).—Gentleman inclines the body without bend of knee, the lady the same, bending the knee raising the r. heel slightly. (2).—Lady glides r.f. backward to 4th position, revolves on it and rise again. (3).—Both draw the front foot to front 3rd position.

1 *bar*. Gentleman goes back with l.f., lady with r.f. to 4th position, dégagé and

1 *bar*. Repeat same step forward with stretched leg en l'air and make a quarter-turn facing each other and finish in 1st position.

2 *bars*. Both; gentleman to left, lady to right, step sideways, the other foot following for a further révérence; the hands are dropped.

2 *bars*. Both turn—gentleman to right, lady to left with one step sideways, returning to the starting point. Hands are again joined.

(1). INTRODUCTION. *Leading out the Lady.*

2 *bars*. Both with r.f. make the *Forward pas.*

2 *bars*. Lady repeat. Gentleman simultaneously make the *Pas to the right*: with these two pas they turn round one another, changing places, gentleman back to the audience, lady facing audience.

4 *bars*. Dropping the hands, they separate with two *Pas to the right,* then gradually retiring towards the place required for the principal figure Z and completing the same whilst they

4 *bars*. Execute the *Pas to the left* (twice).

THE FIGURE Z.

12 *bars*. This figure is completed by two *forward pas en passant*. A better term for this would have been *traversé obliqué.*

12 *bars*. *Pas to the right* (double) and *Pas to the left* repeated in the same sequence three times.

2 *bars*. Balancé and raise r. arms and hands,

6 *bars*. Which they join (*tour des mains*) executing three *forward pas,* then

4 *bars*. With a *Pas to the right* (double) gradually return to the principal figure, the right hand gradually falls back to the original place.

2 *bars*. Balancé and raise l. arms and hands,

6 *bars*. Which they join (*tour des main*) executing three *forward pas,* then

4 *bars*. With a *Pas to the right* (double) retiring gradually to the principal figure the l. hand returns to its original place.

4 *bars*. *Pas to the left.*

12 *bars*. The Principal Figure with two *forward pas* (*traversé*) making

12 *bars*. The *Pas to the right* (double) and the

12 *bars*. *Pas to the left* is repeated three times

THE FINALE.

2 *bars*. Balancé and preparatory raising of both arms and hands,

4 *bars.*   Which they join while doing two *Forward pas* with which they arrive at their original places facing each other and then (the gentleman on the right, lady on the left),

2 *bars.*   Make a *pas sideways* (this time the lady to the left, gentleman to right, returning to the point where the Menuet began.

8 *bars.*   Two révérences, the second one ending the Menuet. Conducting the lady to her seat follows as a matter of courtesey.

Avoid the constant bowing which is seen when the Menuet is danced by amateurs or taught by novices. There should be only the bows at the beginning and end of the dance. Ignorance has inserted bows where the teacher's invention or knowledge failed.

Magny, in his " Choreography " mentions " Menuet Dauphin," " Minuet de la Reine," and " Menuet d'Exaudet," the steps of these are more complex than those of the " Menuet de la Cour."

Menuet de la Cour.—By Perin. Eighty-eight bars, 3-4 tempo. Introduction 10 bars. For the first bar the gentleman takes off his hat; coupé to prepare; pass-pied to face each other; coupé sideways inclining to each other; coupé en arrière in turning, give the hand; passe-pied; coupé en arrière to place; gentleman assemblé l.f. to 3rd rear, lady remaining with her r.f. en avant.

First Part.   Figure 1.   Pas grave (2 bars); assemblé facing each other, coupé, raise r. heel without displacing toe (1 bar); balancé en arrière; coupé à droite; pas de bourrée devant and derrière; coupé en arrière; assemblé pose derrière (3 bars) in all 6 bars.

Figure 2.   Pas grave; pas de menuet turning (4 bars); two pas de menuet to the right (4 bars); coupé, pirouette, coupé en arrière (the gentleman puts his hat on); rond de jambe, three pas marché noble, assemblé devant (4 bars) in all 12 bars.

Figure 3.   1 bar passes. Coupé en arrière r.f.; battement dessus et dessous with l.f; repeat this four times with different foot and épaulement in going backward (4 bars) pas Marcel; coupé to side; balancé en arrière (3 bars) in all 8 bars.

Figure 4.   Pas grave and prepare to present r. hand; three pas marchés; assemblé devant; coupe r.f., present r. hands (4 bars) passe-pied en avant; passe-pied en arrière; passe-pied en arrière; coupé en arrière; assemblé posé en arrière (4 bars) in all 8 bars.

Figure 5.   Pas grave, prepare left hand; three pas marchés assemblé devant, coupé r.f. and, giving l. hand (4 bars) passe-pied en avant, passe-pied en arrière, passe-pied en avant, coupé en arrière, assemblé posé (4 bars) in all 8 bars. The dancers are now vis-a-vis about four paces distant.

Second Part.   Figure 6.   Balancé royal (2 bars) three pas marchés, assemblé en avant, plié (2 bars); **pas de menuet**

to the right, plié, half step of menuet en avant, half step of menuet to the left (4 bars) pas de bourrée derrière et devant; face the corner, coupé en arrière, return to partner with two pas marchés; coupé en arrière, pirouette, pirouette, changing the feet and temps levé (4 bars) in all 12 bars.

Figure 7. Let 1 bar pass. Glissade derrière to the left with épaulement; temps levé; repeat three times with different foot, temps levé, chassé à trois pas facing the corner (4 bars) attitude détournée (marking the time with right heel and pivoting on l. sole) demi-balancé royal; coupé en arrière; assemblé posé derrière (3 bars) in all 8 bars.

Figure 8. Pas grave, prepare to present both hands, three pas marchés approaching partners and returning to original places; assemblé en avant facing each other; coupé de coté (to the side) (4 bars); coupé withdrawing r.f., coupé sideward, present the hands crossed, balancé; pas de bourrée derrière et devant holding hands; coupé en arrière releasing hand to raise the hat; assemblé posé derrière for the gentleman while the lady slowly places r.f. en avant (4 bars) in all 8 bars.

Coda:—Repeat introduction.

Theory of the Steps by Perin. (1) *Coupé*, make an ordinary coupé to face the lady for the salute. (2).—Passe-pied, make some petits battements devant and derrière (*devant* means in front, *derrière* means to the rear) facing the lady. (3).—*Coupé de côté*, make a glissé chassé to the side and salute. (4).—*Pas grave*, glisser r.f. en avant, same with l.f. to the left and assemblé r.f. front. Repeat en arrière (2 bars). (5, 6, 7,) *Balancé*, glissé l.f. en arrière balancing the body to the right, bring r.f. close to l.f., glisé l.f., then raise r.f. devant and derrière, chassé l.f. with r.f. and assemble r.f. rear of l.f. (3 bars). (8).—*Pas de Menuet en tournant*, glissé r.f. to 4th rear position, cross l.f. in front of r.f. and pivot on the soles. Repeat the whole (2 bars). (9).—*Pas de Menuet de côté a droite et à gauche* (4 bars), glissé r.f. to 2nd position bending the knees, glissé point of l.f. to 4th front, s'énlever (raise oneself) slightly on the point of r.f. without moving l.f. (1 bar). Repeat this, commencing l.f. and repeat the whole. (10).—*Pas noble*, pass r.f. to 4th front, then 4th rear, bring l.f. near the r.f. (assemblé), s'énlever on the soles. (11).— Epaulements, when a battement is made with l.f. the right shoulder must be " efface " (turned sideward) and vice-versa. (12).—*Balancé royal*, glisser l.f. en avant oblique, pass r.f. crossed in front, balancé the body en arrière turning the head and shoulders to the right with the bust inclined backward and elevating the right hand forward (1 bar). Repeat to rear (1 bar). (13).—*Demi pas de Menuet*, the legs must be crossed then glide l.f. en avant and assemblé r.f. in front of l.f. (14).—*Temps levé*, s'enlever on the two feet leaving the floor and pass the rear foot to the front. (15).—*Glissade derrière à gauche du pied droit*, these old glissades of the Menuet are made by gliding r.f. behind the left croisé (crossed) the r. heel must be on the left side, r. leg plié (bent) and l. leg stretched, then bring back l.f. gliding it assemblé behind the r.f. (16).—*Chassé à trois pas*, raise r.f. to 2nd en làir, chassé l.f. with the r.f., the foot is then raised obliquely forward. Repeat with l.f., then with r.f. (17).—*Attitude détournée*, the r. arm curved upward, glissé l.f. 4th rear without moving r.f., then raise r. heel and 'pivot on sole of r.f., only the r. heel describes a half-circle while the r. heel marks three beats on the floor, glisser again l.f. to 4th rear without moving r.f. and mark the time with r. heel as before and assemblé l.f. to rear of r.f.

Menuet de la Reine.— Danced by four couples. (1) Salute to the " vis-a-vis." Same to your lady (4 bars). (2).—Make your lady turn under your right arm (2 bars). Salute to your lady (2 bars). (3).—A turn of the hands, right, left, salute (8 bars). (4).—Four " pas de Menuet vis-a-vis " the lady to the left, same the ladies to the gentlemen on the right and assemblé (4 bars). Make that lady turn under your right arm and salute (4 bars). (5).—Repeat these eight last bars with your lady (8 bars). (6).—Repeat these 16 bars. (7).—The four ladies give each other the right hand and make a turn of the left hand with the 1st gentleman, they again give each other the right hand and repeat the turn of the hand with all the gentlemen (32 bars). (8).—Repeat the 4th (8 bars). (9).—Repeat the 5th (8 bars). (10).—The gentlemen turn round their ladies, stop in front of them and salute. Same with all the ladies (16 bars). (11).—The gentlemen salute the ladies on the left, then their own lady, then the vis-a-vis, then their own ladies (8 bars). Finale.—(8 bars) to reconduct their ladies to seats.

Menuet d'Exaudet.—The Menuet d'Exaudet, sung and danced in 1769, was reconstructed in 1893 by Desrat, with the text of the words and the author's choreography. The words are extracted from Favart's comedy, " La Rosière de Solènes " and the choreography from the clever dancing master Exaudet, to whom the music is assigned. Exaudet, born in Rouen about 1710, was in the opera, violin private teacher of the dance in 1749; he composed and made the Menuet on the 25th October, 1769, to which he gave his name. This Menuet obtained such success that it was danced at the court, after having been danced at the theatre and from there, leapt into the " salons " of that time, for a long time it rivalled the Menuet de la Cour, composed by Vestris.

Theory: For a gentleman and a lady:—

1st Part. (16 bars). *Traversé.* Gentleman and lady advance holding each other by the hand, they separate to right and to left, recede in order to face the place where they have started. Then they turn, the gentleman marching behind his lady and stopping in order to salute each other.

2nd Part. (16 bars). The same movements are repeated to return to their original places.

3rd Part. (12 bars). Solo. Alone, the gentleman directs himself to his right and stops; then he directs himself to his left and stops. The lady, after him, directs herself to her left, stops; she begins again to her right and stops. Both draw closer and give each other the two hands.

4th Part. (16 bars). Balancé. Giving both hands to each other, they elevate to the right, to the left, to the right and stop on the tips. Releasing the hands, they make " chassé croisé " to the right moving farther apart from each other; they slowly draw closer and make a turn of the hand to return to their places and salute each other.

5th Part. (12 bars). Balancé. Placing themselves in front of each other, they separate, and draw closer to give each other the hand and return to their places.

6th Part. (16 bars). Traversé. Same movements as in the first part.

7th Part. (16 bars). Retour. Same movements as in the second part.

Menuet Imperial.—Crompton.

Menuet Valse.—1892. Crompton.

Métoecies.—Grecian yearly festival given in honour of the union of the twelve villages of Attica.

Mignon (MIN-YON).—1895. Crompton.

Mimes (MEEM).—The name given in antiquity to the dancers who represented an action, either theatrically, privately, by gestures or in following a deetermined measure accompanied by chants or singing. The first " mimes " are far from offering a very attractive image; not only were they deprived from any instruction and good manners, but the more often rudeness, foolishness and indecency were the only object of their parts. They presented themselves to the public with heads shaven, bare feet, the faces smeared with soot, the body being covered with an animal's skin roughly adjusted. The Romans had two kinds of " mimes," the " mimi-urbani " or public mimes, and the " mimi domestici " or private mimes. The first sometimes held the name of " planipedes," because they danced with naked feet. In his second satire, Horace gives us to understand that women mixed with the mimes, but very rarely. In France, the mimes were suppressed by the order of a Council in the middle ages.

Moelleux.—This adjective is very often employed in the dancing lesson and serves to express the greatest suppleness in every part of the body. A " moelleux " (mellow) dancer does not betray any strain in his step, however be their vigour or their difficulty. Vestris in his time, Genée in our time, are in this respect models to follow.

Moemacteries.—Name of dancers and festivities of Greeks consecrated to Jupiter; they were annual and very much observed by the people.

Mollosika.—Ancient Greek dance of simple easy execution.

Monter (MORN-TAY).—To walk upward to back of stage. *See* Descendre.

Montferine (la).—Italian dance formerly in favour with the Milanese. Simple and elegant, it somewhat resembled the " bourrées " of the Poitou. A gentleman and a lady, sometimes a second gentleman, took part in the dance consisting in " promenades," " ronds " and " tours des mains." When a second gentleman came to join the second, he deprived him of his lady and began again with her the " promenades," " ronds and turn of the hand"; the first gentleman returned to his seat.

Montferine (la).—Italian dance, 1850. 3-4 tempo. Style of bourrée danced by the " Milanese," ladies who, for its execution, have two gentlemen. At times she makes a " promenade " with one of them and makes some " tours de mains " with the other, right hand, left hand, and with the two hands, then, she gives the hand to both gentlemen making them pass under her arms one after the other, then turns on herself without releasing the hands of the gentlemen, then, she takes with her one of the dancers, for the promenade, while the other dances alone imitating the actions of the dancing couples.

Montferine.—Another, 1802. The Montferine is a " bourrée," to which the Milanese ladies, with their sparkling looks, their graceful necks, supple waists, light steps and waving arms, endow with an exquisite charm.

The dance is executed with " promenade " round the salon. All the dancers give each other the hands in a circle, and galop round, then " a tour de mains " gentleman and lady, and it is started again.

Montgolfier (la).—Name of an ancient " contredanse " (quadrille) towards the end of the XVIIIth century, its name was given as being an actuality and was rather general. at public balls.

Morisco.—*See* Morris.

Morisque (la) or **Moresque.**—By the Moors of Spain, 1502. 2-4 tempo. To the sound of trumpets and flutes, the dancers attached small bells to the feet and hands; they were armed and executed some movements of going too and fro, knocking with a foot after each measure to accompany the musicians, then tramping the feet in place and agitating the arms. It made its introduction in Paris, in 1517; but was only danced by burlesque and masked people.

Morphosmos.—Grecian dance mentioned by Athene, as imitating the gestures of animals; it was danced and sung at the same time.

Morris Dance.—The Fools' Dance paved the way for the Morris Dance, which had its origin with the Moors in the Morisco— Morris is a corruption of Moorish. There has been a revival of Morris Dancing in England for some years and the full description of the dances may be found in Mr. Cecil J. Sharpe's books (published by Novello). The dancers were—

the hobby horse (performed by a man) the dragon, Maid Marian, Robin Hood, Friar Tuck, Little John, and the fools Scarlet and Stokesley; they were dressed in the fashions of Edward III. (1216).

Moscovite (la).—Ancient French contredanse. It was a pot-pourri, composed of figures from various dances and executed by any number of couples ad lib.

Moucheter or **Moucheté** (MOOSH-TAY).—*See* " Petits battements," which is the modern technical term.

Moulin (MOO-LAN).—*See* Moulinet.

Moulinet (MOO-LIN-NAY).—Technical term expressing a figure in which several persons, crossing the same hand over each other's, join with the one opposite and move round in the same direction. The word means " a mill," hence " Moulin " or " Moulinet " means the joining of hands to form a mill; ladies moulinet is a ladies' mill; gentlemen's moulinet, gentlemen's mill; grand moulin gentlemen's or ladies' hands joined in centre and holding partner with the other hand. Compare second part of third figure of Lancers. The moulinet figure is pretty general in square dances. Other names for the figure are Chevaux de bois, Double-Chaine, La Croix, The Cross, Tourniquet, etc. The most general are moulinet for four persons. *Demi-moulinet* is when the four opposite dancers with r. hands joined, move round a half-circle.

Movement.—A combination of steps. Action. The teacher often expresses " give more movement to the dance," implying that the pupil should display more life, fire and passion to the dance. In music, the word applies to measure as a " movement in 2-4, or 3-4, " and accompanied by a qualifying term as " quick or slow."

Munychiennes.—Greek dance consecrated to Diana celebrated with great pomp in public places.

N

Nage, *pas de* (NAHJH). Swimming step. From the Greek. While bending both knees glide r.f. to 2nd, hop on r.f. while raising l.f. to 2nd position en l'air, hop on r.f. crossing l.f. rear of r.f., hop on l.f. and assemblé r.f. rear of l.f. While making the first plié (bend of knees) the two arms should be stretched out to the right side to imitate swimming on the side, the arms to the other side for the left movement.

107

Napolitaine, *la.*—Neapolitan dance of the tarantelle order. It is astonishing to find such a rapid dance among a nation proverbially so indolent. The dance consists of rapid small pas serrés (better known as pas bourrées) to 6-8 time.

Nationale, *la,* (NAH SEE-OH-NAHL). A valse carrée or waltz square dance invented by Edward Leblanc of London. Is composed of five figures, the dancers standing in a square. Was first presented at St. James's Hall. Is now obsolete.

Natural (*pas*). (NAH-TOO-RAHL). Another name for *pas marché*.

Navette (*pas de la*) (NAH-VET). Literally to wobble. Any motion of swaying the body to and fro.

Nemesis.—Ancient Grecian dance in honour of the victory of Marathon.

Neurobates.—Ancient "rope dancers" who often executed most difficult steps on the tight-rope.

Nibadismos.—Ancient Grecian comic dance imitating the leaping of goats.

Niobe.—Ancient Grecian dance, also called Daphné, representing the metamorphosis of Daphné.

Noces.—Ancient Greek dances held during nuptial festivities and giving a pretext for excessive libations and debauch. The dancing, which was done by hired dancers, became so licentious that professional dancers were exiled by order of the senate.

Nonime.—This word is employed in ancient French quadrilles to explain the operation of exchanging places with the vis-a-vis and turning backs to each other in doing so. It has long since disappeared from technical dancing terms. The movement was made with glissés-chassés and passing round the vis-a-vis back to back, thus changing places. The figure is an oval and known as *aller et retour* (go on one side and return on the other).

Nymphai.—Ancient Grecian pastoral dance.

Nyssia.—Grecian sacred dance in honour of Bacchus.

Oklasma.—Ancient Greek private dance done with strongly bended knees.

O

Olivettes.—French village dance, somewhat resembling "farandole." The dancers are covered from head to foot with flowers and foliage. Winding in and out among trees and singing they run on until they stop from sheer exhaustion.

One-Step.—A popular modern dance in 2·4 tempo. It is done by walking an ordinary step—two steps to one bar of music. These steps are done in every conceivable direction, forward, backward, sideward or turning. A variation is the "crab-step" which is done by taking (1) one step l.f. sideward, (2) one step r.f. backward, (3) one step l.f. sideward, (4) one step r.f. obliquely forward—lady does the counterpart with the other foot. Dancers insert many of their own variations into the dance, such as, an occasional chassé, a pas marché one step to the bar, the corté of the tango, etc. The appropriate music is "ragtime."

Opposées Rondes (OPPOZAY RAUND) or *rondes opposées.* Opposed circles. The four ladies (in a square dance) advance to the centre, face partners and join hands. They will now be back to back in circle. Gentleman advance two steps and join hands in an outer circle. All now move round to the left. As they are turned toward each other this will make an opposite movement which is very pleasing.

Opposition.—The contrast in the carriage of the members of the body which should be in perfect harmony as in opposition between the foot and arm. This is based on the natural walk in which the movements of the feet and arms are by nature opposed to each other. Opposition requires also the assistance of the head, shoulders and hips. In every sideward movement the raising of the arm and turn of the head is always contrary to the side where the movement is made. In bending movements, the arms should be raised; in rising, the arms must be lowered. In moving to the right the arms should go to the left and vice versa. In moving forward the arms should go back and vice versa. Left hand and right foot go forward simultaneously and vice versa. (See Bras, port de).

Oranges and Lemons.—Old English Country Dance in Quadrille form. (Figure 1). All advance to centre and retire twice, gentlemen bowing to partners and to vis-a-vis. Gentlemen advance to centre (moulinet), join hands and go half-round into opposite places. Ladies bow to left and right, join hands in centre, go half-round and join partners opposite. Gentlemen repeat and ladies repeat, this will take all back to places. (Figure 2). All form two lines, advance and retire. Take partner's r. hand go round each other four steps; change hand and repeat. Lady go to next gentleman, gentleman to next lady and repeat until places are regained. (Figure 3). Partners link arms and go round each other twice; first and second couples take hands and walk half-round while the third and fourth bow elaborately to each other; first and second couple go half-round, third and fourth go half-round. Then first and last couples bow to each other while second and third couple go half-round simultaneously and in so doing regain original places.

Orchesography.—The Art of writing steps and gestures. This science preceded our choreography and the first treatise on the subject was published by a Canon of Langres named Thoinot Arbeau in 1588 under the pseudonym Jean Tabourot. Several masters wrote books on this Art, among them Feuillet, Beauchamps, Magny, Saint-Léon. An incomparable work on the subject is that by Frederick Zorn of Odessa, whose precious book has been translated into many languages. (See Choreography).

Ordinaire (*pas*), Ordinary field step, 112 to 116 steps a minute : a quicker step is pas accelleré or quick step, 144; slower, is parade step, 70 a minute.

Origin of the word " Dance." It is derived from the Arabic " Tanza " which means the favourite exercise of ladies. In German it is " Tanz"; Spanish, " Danca "; Italian, " Danza "; French, " Danse "; Greek, " Sikelizeo." It is also termed " Saltation," from the Latin " Saltare," adjective " Saltatory " which means leaping, or used in leaping. The Muse or Goddess of the Dance is " Terpsichore," derived from " Terpo," I charm, and " Choros," dance.

Orobates.—The rope-dancers of Greece who, according to ancient authors, possessed surprising ability and audacity in their dancing.

Orsites.—Crete dance mentioned by Athene.

Ortense.—The ortense is the flowering hydrangea from a single stem of which many thousands of small flowrets are sent forth. This name is therefore used for a multiplicity of caprioles.

Ostrich Dance of the natives of Africa imitating the movements of Ostriches.

Oula.—The dance of some of the Oceania Islands.

Ouvert (oo-VAIR).—Any movement in which the legs are open sideways to right or left. (See Ouverture).

Ouverture (oo-VER-TOOR).—Keeping the legs apart in dancing. The teacher frequently employs the expression " ouverture des jambes " (opening the legs) meaning to ask the pupil to turn the knees outward or technically " en dehors," the sine qua non of the good dancer.

P

Paeoniennes.—Grecian feasts danced in honour of Apollo, they were also sacred

Palestrique.—The " polestrique" with the Greeks was more a "gymnastic " than a dance; it comprised the exercises of wrestling, boxing, racing, jumping, throwing of the " disc and the hoop", however there existed between it and Saltation a great simi-larity, applying all the exercises of suppleness, force and vigour.

Pamperke.—This dance also called "pampenuque," was used in Bayonne; it was composed of circles and of passes. The men were decorated with ribbon of all colours and conducted by one ot them whom they nominated "king of the feast." Gentleman and lady dancers of equal number accompanied by the sound of the flute hold each other by a long ribbon, and encircle the king who directs them with a stick raised above his head. From time to time a couple come out and turn in front of the joyful "monarch," then resume their place in the ring; another succeeds them, and so on. At the end of the dance the king chooses a lady, and lifts the ribbon, ot which they each hold an extremity. All the dancers pass alternately under this ribbon, marching four by four.

Panathénées.—Great feasts and religious dances instituted by Lycurgus in honour of Apollo; they have been found on Ancient Grecian monuments; and were celebrated sometimes in the temples, sometimes on the public highways.

Pantalon.—This word signified in the middle ages a jester dancer executing the "danses Sautés." In 1830, the first figure of our quadrille was called thus, which was primitively called "chaîne Anglaise." The author ot a new music seized for a title an actuality which created a great sensation at the court balls. For the first time, trousers were seen to be substituted for the short breeches, and the author stigmatized this fact by giving this name of "pantalon" to the first figure. For fuller details see "Quadrille."

Pantomime and Pantomimes.—These two words find their explanation in their Grecian etymology: representing everything by gestures, that is to say: to mimic instead of speaking; to pourtray by the movements of the members of the body alone all actions, facts, ideas, sentiments, and passion. The "pantomimes" then, were the representatives of this art which attained such a high esteem with the ancients. These dancers, also often authors, enjoyed such favour in Rome that they more than once created some embarrassment to the governors in the days of political convulsions. Their part and importance permitted them rather large licence. The science of these pantomimes had to be very deep, since Cassiodore says that it consisted in representing to nature, the pourtrayal by gesture, steps, and attitudes, all the actions of men, without the help of words, they should have been as eloquent as the greatest orators; Cassiodore ironically adds: "and more intelligible than they were."

The pantomime dances were called after the names of heroes or ot the gods whose lives were represented. Primitively the dancers were accompanied by comical or tragical authors who sang and danced; later, they figured alone. In the reign of Augustus, we find the first great pantomimes really worthy of that title; we owe to them the creation of the danced theatrical action, which produced our most celebrated masters of ballet. Pylades and Bathylle have left in the history of dances the germ of the art of Gardel and Dauberval. Outside of their service at the theatre, these pantomimes were often called in at the feasts, weddings and family parties. Juvenal speaks of one of these dancers, as a carver at table, and makes us believe that in his time, the functions of mimes were multiplied, for not only did the dancer carve the dishes with art, but at each course he executed a dance.

The debauch of the Roman women brought damage to the prestige of the pantomimes and drew upon them the attention of the public. Already scenes of rivalry between the two great masters had given cause for troubles at the theatre and in the town, and it is then that the Emperor Trojan was forced to expel them from Rome. All these mimes had positions sufficiently lucrative to acquire considerable fortunes, despite the luxurious lives which they led.

A part of the word " pantomime," we find synonymous words in several authors, " artifices," " chironomie," " chiron-autes," " chresophi," " petaminarii," " apolausti," " orchisae," " hypocritae," " gesticulatores," " ethopoces." These names are evidently derived either from their own character, or from their general attribute. It is certain that there were women mimes making profession of this art.

The lady mime dancers of Cadiz were celebrated in antiquity by the infinite and irresistible art which they displayed in captivating the spectators. Their dance was divided in three parts, 1st the " chironomie," actions of the hands; 2nd, " l'halma," actions of the feet; 3rd, " l'altissima," action of the elevated jumps. Many poets were unable to find expressions strong enough to paint the voluptuousness which these pantomimists inspired in dancing! According to Lucien, in his " Diologue de la danse," the mimes changed clothes when changing parts and took care to wear costumes appropriate to the personages whom they represented. They wore the tunic and the " palla," the stole, the " talaris," a sort of short tunic, and the " syrma," a long drapery usually worn by the courtezans. Several of them adopted for effective parts the coquus," large lined garment, the mytre, the tiara and the ridisniculum with head ornament for women. The " toge " was prohibited but the mask was imperative.

Parisian Quadrille.—Danced the same as Quadrille but in two lines instead of a square.

Parisienne, by Giuseppe Galimberti ; Milan 1898. 8 bars of 2/4.

A round dance for one couple. Gentleman and lady place themselves one in front of the other vis-a-vis. They give each other the right hand to the right hand and left hand to left hand, placing their hands in form of a cross. In this position they start off both with the right foot in making 4 pas marchés in the style of a " tour de main gauche " (turn of left hand) alternating the foot for two measures. Repeat these 2 measures starting with the left foot and in turning to the right.

Then they release hands and the gentleman's right takes the left hand of the lady, and place himself on a same line (position of the pas-de-quatre).

They make 2 " pas marchés " en avant for 1 measure, they change hands facing " en arrière " and make 2 other " pas marchés " for 1 measure, then they clasp round each other in order to execute quickly, two " tours de valse sautée rapide " (or boston). Repeat, ad lib.

Pas. Theoretically one calls "pas" (step) the union of several " temps " or movements of the feet. At the theatre, this word takes another meaning and signifies the harmony of a dance executed by several dancers. One says " pas de quatre " or " pas de deux '' or " pas de six."

Anciently, the theory of pas was quite different, and implied the idea of a single movement of the foot, consequently, was confused with the word " temps," which must be used, for a step or pas is a composition of " temps." On this subject, the Diderot " Encyclopaedia " gives the following theory of the steps taken in its ancient meaning. The five steps are different:—1st, the " pas droit," which is made in a straight line; 2nd, the " pas grave," or open, which is made " en écartant " (opening the legs) while walking, a foot of the other and in describing a semi-circle; 3rd, the " pas battu," so called when one of the legs is passed over or passed under the other, before placing the foot to the ground, or again when the thighs are knocked against each other; 4th the " pas tourné," when by a " tour des jambes," a full circle is described with the foot " en avant " or " en arrière "; it is also called " tour de jambes "; 5th, the " pas tortillé," when a foot is made to move on a line parallel to the one which is placed on the ground, and that when placing it to the ground, it is replaced at right angles; the step, in one word, is " tortillé " when, in starting the tip of the foot is turned inward and, in placing it, it is turned again outward, the hip then takes part in the movements and facilitates its execution by the " dehors " (outside) which it possesses. (See Ouverture).

Moreover, the pas of the middle ages, of which Diderot speaks, contained several others used in what were then called " contredanses," which had no connection whatever with our modern pas: the " pas neuf '' or " pas relevé," which was made by raising one's-self after having " plié '' (bent) in the middle of a step; the " pas balancé " or the " balance-ment '' (balancing), when one " se jette " to the right or to the left on the tip of the foot to make then a " coupé "; the " pas coupé," which means when, after having made a pas alerte or only " movementé,'' another slower one is made; the " pas dérobé," when the two feet are moved at the same time in opposite direction; the " pas glissé," when a step is made longer than it should be naturally, as its length is determined by the length of the shoulders; the " pas chassé" or simply " chassé,'' when a " plié " is made before moving the feet in order to " chasser " one " en avant " or " en arrière "; the " pas tombé,'' when a " plié " is made only after having placed the foot which has been put in motion, then the " pas mignardés," which are so called when the movements of the feet follow the time given to the notes of music, as when one converts the five white minims into ten black minims (old expression to convert the "whites" into "blacks."). I have borrowed this long theory from "Alembert's Encyclopædia" to establish the difference of the word " pas " anciently with the sense given to it to-day. This quotation also demonstrates which were the first steps used in ballroom dances.

Pas Bohemian. Step employed in the first polkas, but is since abandoned in the salons ; it is found again in the balls frequented by the military under the name of " pas piqué." This step consisted in tapping the heel on the ground after having stretched the leg, and to lift up again this leg in order to make it execute the " pas de polka." In Poland, Hungary, and in Bohemia, this step is very much used, but the " coup de talon " (knock of the heel) is twice given at the first temps of the measure.

Pas de Danse (un). " Pas de danse " is the name given to the temps which comprise the steps for the dance ; for example:— A " pas de polka " with the right foot ; 1st measure,— two crochets or four quavers for the four movements of this " pas de polka." A " pas de valse " of two measures, six crochets, six " temps " for a complete measure, etc.

The steps of all the dances of the world, either of the salon or of the theatre, may be made to all the measures of music, or moderating or quickening the time. Good ear is necessary for the harmony of the music and the steps.

Pas d'Avant Deux (PAH DAHVAHN DER). See also " Theatre." These movements and dances are usually executed by two or more dancers doing the same steps.

Forty movements known as *Pas d'Avant Deux Civil.* In bars of 2-4 rhythm. These are danced by series of four persons placed as in Quadrille (*vis-a-vis*). The four dancers commence with a *Pas Francais* en avant then *Pas Francais* en arrière, then two more en avant to change places with vis-a-vis and repeat the whole to return to places.

Balancé. Face Partners. Make a pas francais to the right, one to the left, one to change places with partner, and one to return to place. These twelve pas francais will take 24 measures of music. As will be seen these steps are made en avant, en arrière à droit, à gauche, obliquely and en tournant and it is the same with all the steps described.

(1). PÀS FRANCAIS **EN AVANT** and **EN ARRIÈRE** EN AVANT. (1). Glide r.f. forward. (2). Chassé forward. (3). Jeté l.f. forward. (4). Assemblé r.f. in front of l.f. EN ARRIÈRE (1). Glide l.f. to rear. (2). Chassé backward. (3). Jeté r. leg to rear. (4). Assemblé l.f. to rear of r.f.

(2). JETÉ. EN AVANT (2 measures). (1). Jeté r.f. forward. (2). Sauté (hop) on r.f. (3). Jeté on l.f. forward. (4). Assemblé r.f. in front. EN ARRIÈRE (2 measures). (1). Jeté l.f. backward. (2). Hop on l.f. (3). Jeté on r.f. (4). Assemblé.

(3). PAS FRANCAIS à DROIT and à GAUCHE (to right and to left) 4 measures. (1). Glide r.f. to side. (2). Chassé. (3). Coupé. (4). Assemblé r.f. rear of l.f. Reverse for the left.

(4). SISSONNES in *three temps* to left and to right. PIROUETTES to left (4 measures). (1). Sauté (hop) on r.f. keeping l.f. in rear. (2). Sauté on r.f. stretching l.f. to the side. (3). Assemblé l.f. in front of r.f. Reverse to make sissonnes to left. The Pirouettes.—(1). Make a quarter turn to left in gliding l.f. to the rear. (2). Hop on l.f., in making a quarter-turn pass r.f. in front of l.f. (3). Repeat (and) jeté r.f. en arrière. (4). Assemblé l.f. rear of r.f.

(5). SISSONNES in *five temps* to the right and to the left (4 measures). (1). Sauté on l.f. keeping r.f. up in rear. (2). Sauté on l.f. stretching r. leg up at the side. (3). Sauté on l.f. passing r.f. up in front (and) jeté r.f. forward. (4). Assemblé l.f. in front. Reverse for other foot.

(6). FOUETTÉ l.f. rear of r.f. ASSEMBLÉ l.f. front of r.f., pass r.f. rear of l.f., assemblé r.f. in front of l.f., three DEBOITÉS en arrière; jeté and assemblé (4 measures). *Analysis.* (1). Hop on r.f. passing l.f. rear of r.f. (this is known as *coup de mollet* (*coo-der-mollay*), literally, stroke of the calf). (2). Assemblé l.f. in front of r.f. (3). Hop on l.f. and pass r.f. to rear. (4). Assemblé r.f. in front of l.f. (5). Three quick desboités (*see this word*) backward. (6). Jeté r.f. backward. (7). Jeté l.f. backward (and) jeté r.f. backward. (8). Assemblé l.f. rear of r.f.

(7). DÉGAGÉ right foot to the side to pass it devant (*before*) and derrière (*rear*) of the left, jeté and assemblé (2 measures). (1). Sauté on l.f. gliding r.f. to the side. (2). Sauté twice on l.f. while passing r.f. back and front of l.f. (3). Jeté r.f. forward. (4). Assemblé l.f. in front. Reverse for the other foot.

(8). PAS CHEVAL à droite (2 measures). (1). Stretch r. leg horizontally to side. (2). Sauté on l.f. and glissé r.f. to right side. (3). Chassé (and) jeté r.f. forward. (4). Assemblé l.f. in front. Reverse for the other leg.

(9). SISSONNES in front in *five temps* (2 measures). (1). Make three sautés on l.f. while passing r.f. in front of l.f. (2). Stretch out r. leg to side and pass it to rear. (3). Jeté r. leg forward. (4). Assemblé l.f. in front, Reverse for the other leg.

(10). ÉCHAPPÉ en avant, pass l.f. back and before, jeté, assemblé and pirouette. (2 measures). (1). From the 3rd position jump and fall on l.f. with r. leg stretched forward. (2). Dégagé on r.f. and pass l.f. back and front of r.f. (3). Jeté l.f. forward. (4). Assemblé r.f. in front of left turning (see No. 4).

(11). PAS de ZÉPHYR in 8 temps (4 measures). (1). Sauté on r.f. while passing l.f. to rear. (2). Stretch l. leg out in front, hop on r.f. bringing l.f. over r.f. (3). Stretch out lett leg forward and chassé backward. (4). While hopping on l.f., place r.f. over l.f. (5). Stretch r. leg forward and chassé backward. (6). Hop on r.f. with l.f. over it and stretch l. leg forward. (7). Jeté l. leg forward. (8). Assemblé r.f. in front.

(12). CROISADE (Krooah-sahd) to right. (2 measures). (1). Rond de jambe (that is, *round the leg*) the r. leg to r. side (2). Cross l.f. in front of r.f. (and) glissade r.f. to r. side. (3). Cross-chassé l.f. over r.f.—this is *chassez croissé*. (4). Assemblé r.f. in front of l.f. Repeat to the left. (2 measures).

(13). TWO PETITS BATTEMENTS front and back, jeté and assemblé (2 measures). (1). Make two sautés on l.f. while passing r.f. twice in front of l.f. (2). Sauté on l.f. passing r.f. to rear. (3). Jeté r.f. forward. (4). Assemblé l.f. in front. Repeat for the other foot (2 measures).

(14). GRAND BATTEMENT to the right (2 measures). (1). Stretch up r. leg to r. side. (2). Sauté on l.f. bringing r. foot over l.f. (3). Sauté on l.f. stretching r. leg up again. (4). Assemblé r.f. rear of l.f. Repeat for the other leg (2 measures).

(15). FOUR GRANDS BATTEMENTS. Same as the preceding, four times (4 measures).

(16). TOMBÉ ('tombay; fall) in 5 temps (2 measures). (1). Sauté on r.f. while stretching l. leg to l. side. (2). Cross l.f. behind r.f., chassé r.f. to r. side. (3). Fall back on l.f. and stretch r. leg to r. side and bring it to rear (and) jeté r.f. en avant. (4). Assemblé l.f. in front.

(17). TOMBÉ in 3 temps, POINTÉ de TALON (to mark with the heel) DE LA POINTÉ and assemblé (4 measures). (1). Stretch l.f. to left side and put it down close to r.f., raising r.f. (2). Tombé (fall) on r.f. (3). Cross l.f. behind r.f. and chassé, raising r. leg to side. (4). Assemblé r.f. to rear. (5). Sauté on l.f. and point the heel of r.f. to the side. (6). Sauté on l.f. and point the toe of r.f. to r. side. (7). Sauté on l.f. (8). Assemblé r.f. in front.

(18). JETÉ en avant, three CHANGEMENTS DES TALONS (changes of heels), JETE en arrière and three CNANGEMENTS DES TALONS (4 measures). (1). Jetè r.f. en avant. (2). Jeté l.f. en avant (and) Sauté on l.f. stretching r. leg to the side (3-4). Three changes of the feet—the first is assemblé, then jump and change the feet twice. Repeat this making the jetés backward.

(19). POINTÉ SISSONNE, pointer du talon, de la pointe à côté, assemblé en avant, sissonne en avant (4 measures). (1). Sauté on l.f. pointing heel of r.f. at the side with well-stretched leg. (2). Sauté on l.f. pointing toe of r.f. at side. (3). Sauté on l.f. and assemblé r.f. to 3rd front. (4). Sauté on l.f., bringing r.f. over and in front of l.f. (5). Sauté on l.f. stretching r. leg to r. side. (6). Sauté on l.f. and assemblé r.f. in 3rd rear (7-8) Pause.

(20). GRANDS BATTEMENTS TOMBÉ, a grand battement to the right, assemblé, tombé in three temps to the right (2 measures). (1). Sauté on l.f. stretching r. leg up to r. side. (2). Sauté on l.f. and pass r.f. in front of l.f., the tip of r.f. touching tip of l.f. (3). Sauté on l.f. and assemblé r.f. to 3rd rear and tombé in three temps to the right (see step 17).

(21). JETÉ EN AVANT and ENTRECHAT, same en arrière (4 measures). (1). Jeté r.f. en avant keeping l.f. in rear. (2). Jeté l.f. en avant (and) sauté on l.f. and stretch r. leg up to right side. (3). Assemblé r.f. in front of l.f. (4). Entrechat. *Analysis of Entrechat.* Bend both knees, spring upwards as high as possible with both legs quite straight and the toes pointed downward, make the calves touch each other, and in the spring, change the feet twice, *i.e.*, cross and re-cross, finishing with r.f. in front. Coming down with feet together is *tombé assemblé.* For this step en arrière, make the jeté backward.

(22). ZÉPHYR of left leg, jeté, assemblé and pirouette to left (4 measures). (1). Sauté on r.f. raising l.f. in rear and then stretch out l.f. en avant. (2). Jeté l.f. en avant (and) sauté on l.f. stretching r. leg to the side. (3). Assemblé r.f. in front of l.f. (4). Pirouette to the left (see step 4).

(23). CHASSÈ, PÀS de BOURRÉE, JETÉ and ASSEMBLÉ, to the right and left (4 measures). (1). Stretch out the r. leg forward and chassé backward. (2). Three pas de bourrée en avant. (*Analysis of pas de bourrée*). After the chassé the l. leg will be stretched up in the rear; glisser l.f. under r.f. three times (*coupé dessous*) rising on the sole of r.f. which makes three small sautés glissés en avant, the l.f. making three small chassés under r.f.) (3). Jeté r.f. en avant and assemblé r.f. in front.

(24). PAS RUSSE (same as *pas de basque*) en avant, two PIROUETTES VOLANTES to right. The pirouette volante (*flying pirouette*) is known also as *pirouette anglaise.* (1). Rond de jambe the right leg (round the right leg) to the side (and) glide l.f. forward. (2). R.F. to 3rd rear (3-4). Repeat commencing with l.f. (5 to 8) two pirouettes volantes in which two complete turns are made. (*Analysis of pirouette volante, or anglaise*). The r.f. is placed 4th rear, tip of l.f. is crossed in front of r.f. and, rising on both toes, make a complete turn; or, rond de jambe r. leg to 4th rear, place tip of l.f. close to rear and well crossed, rise on the tips and make a complete turn.

(25). DÉGAGÉ ENTRECHAT, open the EQUERRE (square) without marking the time, ASSEMBLÉ, ÉCART and ENTRECHAT (4 measures). (1) Petit dégagé r.f. to r. side; (2) Entrechat r.f. in front of l.f.; (3) and in falling back (retombé) assemblé r.f. to rear (4, 5, 6). Repeat this beginning l.f. (*and*) equerre without marking time (that is, rise and pivot on the soles while turning and opening out the heels, then put the heels down, pivot on them and open out the toes (7) assemblé r.f. in front (*and*) écart

117

en l'air (throw the legs wide in the air, that is with a spring) and entrechat finishing l.f. in front.

(26) PETIT DÉGAGÉ or r.f. to right side, CHANGEMENTS DES TALONS (heels), same with the other foot, EQUERRE and three CHANGEMENTS DES TALONS (pronounced *tah-law*) (4 measures). (1). Sauté on l.f. while making dégagé of r.f. to r. side. (2). Changements des talons commencing with r.f. in front (3, 4). Repeat with other foot. (5). Equerre. (6). Equerre. (7 and 8) three changements des talons.

(27). POINTER DE LA POINTE of the heel, PETIT BATTEMENTS in front, jeté and assemblé; repeat with other foot (4 measures). Each of these movements has already been described, this enchaînement should therefore be easily followed.

(28). TWO PETITS BATTEMENTS devant and pirouette to left, repeat other foot (4 measures). See note to No. 27.

(29). PAS RUSSE (see No. 24) Pas de bourrée(4 measures). Make (1-4) two pas russes forward (5-7) three pas bourrées to rear. (8). Assemblé.

(30). POINTER in seven temps to right and left (4 measures) (1-7) Sauté on l.f. pointing the other foot heel and toe (and) fouetté (8) assemblé.

(31). CHASSÉ OUVERT en avant, PIROUETTE to left (4 measures). (1). Glisser (glide) r.f. forward to right. (2). Chassé r.f. from its place by l.f. (3). Glisser l.f. to l. side. (4). Chasser l.f. by the r.f. crossing behind. (5). Assemblé l.f. rear of r.f. (6-8) pirouette to the left with grand battement.

(32). TWO PETITS BATTEMENTS in front of each foot, *assemblé* and pirouette to left (4 measures) (1-2). Sauté twice on l.f. passing r.f. twice in front of l.f. (3-4) repeat other foot. (5). Assemblé l.f. rear of r.f. (6-7-8-) pirouette to left with entrechat and assemblé.

(33). CONTRETEMPS SIMPLE to right and to left (4 measures). (1). Glisser r.f. to r. side. (2). Pass l.f. which is raised at rear of r.f. and cross it in front of r.f. (3). Stretch r. leg to right side and make a grand battements of r.f. in front of l.f. (4). Assemblé r.f. to rear. Repeat other foot.

(34). CONTRETEMPS BATTU to right and to left. It is made en brisé and entrechat instead of the simple crossing.

(35). TWO PAS RUSSE en avant, two AILES de PIGEON COUPEES to rear and assemblé (4 measures).

(36). AILES de PIGEON COUPÉS to the side (4 measures).

(37). AILES de PIGEON *simple* (4 measures).

(38). AILES de PIGEON *en tournant* (4 measures).

(39). ÉCART, entrechat and tour en l'air (2 measures). Tour en l'air (pronounced toorahn lair) is a turn in the air, *i.e.*, with both feet off the floor.

(40). AILES de PIGEON terre à terre and attitude (4 measures).

Pas des Patineurs(PAH-TEE-NER) Skating dance. Arranged by Willemot of Paris, 1894. Position: - Stand side by side facing forward, gentleman's r. arm round lady's waist, or join both right hands and both left hands (crossed). *Step* 1. (1). Glissé r.f. to the right. (2). Glissé l.f. well crossed rear of right. (3). Glissé r.f. to the right. (4). Hop on r.f. passing l. leg in front of right leg well stretched (2 bars). Repeat other foot (2 bars). *Step* 2. Going quickly forward and retaining the lady by the waist. (1). Place r. foot en avant. (2). Hop on it passing l. leg forward (3-4). repeat with l. foot (5.6.7.8.). Repeat with right and left foot (4 bars). Repeat step 1 and so on. Variation—without losing the measure, during the second part the gentleman moves to the front of his partner, both make the first step to the right which will separate them, then to the left which will bring them together again. They can also take each other's r. hands and make the second step going round each other. Bend the body to right when going to the left and vice versa.

Pas Plongé.—Imitate a man plunging into the water. Both hands joined, arms stretched forward, lower head and hands, and while raising l. hand very high to the rear, assemblé, imitating a swimmer. Repeat with other hand and foot.

Pas de Quatre.—Dance performed by four persons. A famous pas de quatre was danced by Lucille Grahn, Cerito, Carlotta Grisi and Taglioni.

Pas de Quatre.—By R. M. Crompton, 1890. A round dance.

Pas de Quatre.—See Barn Dance.

Passacaille (PAS-CAH YEH). A dance of XVIII. century favoured at the Court of Louis XIV., and was very solemn and majestic. Chéruel in his "Dictionary" of the habits and customs of France speaks of it only from the musical point of view and compares it to a "chaconne" but with the singing in a more tender strain. Trevoux's "Dictionary" defines it as a dance in 3-4 tempo with gestures and slow movements. In Brossard's "Dictionary of Music" it says: "this dance is a Chaconne, the steps of which are temps of long glissés and stretching the arms to the side, the knees bent slowly on the first temps simultaneously to the arms opening to right and left, on the last two temps one rose again after making a dégagé to the right or left, the arms assuming their natural position." This step was the origin of the "pas de menuet."

Holding partner's hand, the step was "glisser r.f. to 2nd position, assemblé, pirouette, réverence (4 measures). Same for lady but with the other foot.

Passepied (PAHS-PEE-AY). XVII. century, Classed among the Branles (brawls) of Brittany. *The Step.*—Tempo 3-4. (1). Glissé l.f. en avant. (2). Glissé r.f. en avant. (3). Glissé l.f. en avant. (4). Tip of r. toe to l. toe. (5). Tip of r. toe to l. heel. (6). Plié (bend) l. knee and raise r. leg forward (4th

---

elevation) 2 measures for the gentleman, lady same with opposite foot. Repeat, commencing other foot, 2 measure. *Another description.* Join hands facing each other. (1). Both pas de basque to right turning l. shoulder forward, then pas de basque to left turning r. shoulder forward, walk round three steps to change places. (2). Coupé and pas bourrée three times. (3). Jeté r.f. over l.f. and vice versa. (4). Pas de basque diagonally four bars forward and four bars backward. (5). Cross hands and pas de basque backward. (6). Arms round each other's necks and go round with eight pas cheval (pawing the ground like a horse). (7). Make a turn backward with pas de basque and heel shuffle to the right. (8). Repeat same to left. For music, the passepied from Destouches's first opera " Isse " is a good example.

Passepied de la Cour (PAS DU). Tempo 3-4. (1). r.f. to 4th elevation. (2). Tip of r.f. to tip of l.f. (3). Tip of r.f. to heel of l.f. (4). Dégagé on r.f. rear of l.f. (5). Glissé l.f. en avant. (6). Assemblé r.f. to l.f. (2 measures).

Pastorale.—Ancient and Modern pastoral dances. The pastorale was the termination of all Greek dances.

Pastourelle.—The fourth figure of Quadrille (see Quadrille). Before 1830 this figure was danced with the couple *on the left* of the leading couple and not with the couple vis-a-vis. It was sometimes called VILLANELLE.

Patau.—Dance of the savage races of Oceania.

Pavane, Pavan, Pavanne (PAH-VAHN).—The spellings are various—is one of the oldest foreign dances we have, and was the dance of kings, queens, lords, and dames of high degree in the Courts of Italy, Spain, France, and England as far back, it is said, as the thirteenth century. Certainly it was already old when Thoinot Arbeau, the monkish historian of the dance, gave its description, with words and music, in his history of dancing published in 1588; and the one he gives " Belle qui tiens ma vie," is the most in use to-day. Some have traced its derivation to Padua, and make it out a Padovan dance. But the derivation from Pavo, *Pavono,* peacock, is the more acceptable, for the dance itself has all the leisured grace, the noble stateliness of the peacock, the spreading of whose tail the dancers emulate in displaying the trains of their costumes when they tread the measure. Its invention is ascribed to Ferdinand Cortez, the Spaniard. The music in stately 2-4 tempo consisted of two themes of 8 bars each, repeated, making 32 bars in all. Singing accompanied the dance.

1. Begin, side by side, hand in hand, with a curtsey and a bow. Start with a pas marché down the floor, making four steps, the gentleman taking the lady's left hand. They commence with opposite feet. The gentleman holds the lady's right hand *en tour*—that is, they turn with four steps. He then takes her left hand and goes up the floor backwards, with four steps. He again takes her right hand and turns with four steps. This accomplishes the first movement.

2. The gentleman passes the lady from his right to his left in three steps, then they both pose, facing the audience, with the toe pointed. The gentleman passes the lady from the left to his right with three steps, both change hands, and pose in a line facing the audience. The gentleman passes the lady to his left in three steps, when both pose, with their backs to the audience.

All is very slowly performed in stately measure.

3. The lady passes under the left arm of the gentleman, holding hands as they do so, but they loose them when the movement is over. Standing vis-à-vis they take one step to the right and salute, and one step to the left and salute, and then again one step to the right and salute, which means that the man makes a sweeping bow and the lady a very low curtsey.

4. The gentleman passes the lady under his right arm, makes a step to the left, and bows. They then make a step to the right, placing that foot over the left, then carry out the half turn, point left toe to toe, and shoulder to shoulder, in a very graceful pose. This is repeated four times, forming a sort of cross with the feet; the last time, instead of a pose, they salute each other.

An unsuccessful attempt was made in 1844 to revive the dance, but the polka and waltz had then the grip of public favour. The dance in now used only on the stage or for the purposes of pageantry.

The Pavane went through many alterations, and in my collection are descriptions of thirty-three different Pavanes of various periods, but in contradiction to some contemporaries who wrote them in 3-4 time, the originals are written in 2-4 time. Arbeau (1588) writes in his theory of the Pavane, " The movement is " binaire " (2) consisting of a white minim and two black ones." In spite of the embryonic state of Arbeau's choreography it has been possible to faithfully reconstruct the dance and the music.. The original dance and music were reconstructed by Signoret and published by Borneman, (Paris 1886) from the text of Arbeau and may be obtained from Borneman, 2, Rue de l'Abbaye, Paris. Before commencing the dance, the couples promenade round the hall and gravely salute the host; it was sometimes followed by a " Gaillarde" to amuse the spectators. The reconstruction of Pavane: The dance is done to a measure lento in two temps with the following step made sometimes en avant, en arrière, à côté and en tournant. *Pas de Pavane*:—(1) Bend the knees and glissé forward r.f. (2) Stretch l. leg forward, the point of l.f. touching the floor. For the l.f. make the movements with the other foot. For turning, rise on the sole. *Part* 1. Two couples facing each other, describe a large semi-circle to the right and change places, this is pas de pavane to the right, keeping the hands up very high. The two couples salute each other. Repeat to return to places. *Part* 2. Both couples make four pas de pavane advancing to the right and stop, facing each other and salute partners. Two pas de pavane advancing to opposite couple and taking opposite lady's r.

hand, make a tour de main finishing facing own partner. Gentleman's l. hand takes lady's right held high up and return with four pas de pavane to place and salute each other. *Part* 3. One Gentleman alone make a large semi-circle to the left with four pas de pavane and arrived in front of the opposite lady, both salute; he makes another semi-circle to place and salute with partner. The other gentleman repeats. *Coda.* Both couples (without holding hands) go to the right with four pas de pavane and salute vis-a-vis; face partners and salute again, from this point lead partners to seats, or make a promenade round the room as at the beginning.

Pavane (*pas de*). Another description. (1) Glissé l.f. forward. (2) glissé r.f. forward, (3) glissé l.f. forward, (4) raise r.f. to 4th forward elevation. Another. Repeat (1) (2) (3) and for (4), touch point of l.f. with point of r.f. and immediately raise r. leg forward. In 1589 the step was made thus:— " one pas en avant and three en arrière and repeat." In 1604, the Chancellor sent a messenger to the Monsieur Nicholas (Secretary to Henri IV) who was dying, to ask after his health. He replied " Tell Monsieur the Chancellor, that I am as well as the Pavane, one step en avant and three en arrière." In 1515, it was " (1) pas marché en avant, (2-3) two small ones en arrière, (4) elevate a foot forward." In 1547, (1) " Glisser r.f. forward, (2) same l.f., (3) point of r.f. to toe of l.f., (4) raise r.f. forward. Repeat with same foot, three times and at the fourth time assemblé for the fourth beat, and then repeat the whole commencing l.f." The steps of later Pavanes were practically the same.

Pécorée Calabrian dance: derived from *pécora*, a sheep; from *pécore*, a stupid creature; the rapid agitated movements recall the ancient rigaudons. The dancers move their bodies as much as the legs.

Perigourdine. From Perigord. The dancers do some rapid chassés with change of hands to form a chain.

Périn. French Quadrille named after its author Mons Périn of Paris, 1859. At that time the Waltz feverishly absorbed the dancers and this quadrille came as a welcome relief. Each of the five figures was played twice.

Persike. Sacred dance of the Greeks, later found in Persia.

Petit (PET-EE), **Petite** (PET-EET), **Petits** (pl. PET-EE). Small. Movements of the feet when the toe rests on the floor, as *petit* rond de jambe; when raised from the floor they become " *grand.*" *Petit rond* in square dances is the small circle of four persons as in fourth figure of Quadrilles. *Grand rond* is the grand circle made by all the dancers.

Pied de dedans (PEE-AY DER DAY DAHN). Inside foot. **Pied de dehors** (PEE-AY DER DAYOR). Outside foot. In square dances a gentleman advancing to his vis-a-vis and joining r. hands both

will have r. foot inside (*dedans*) and' d.f. will b,e outside
(*dehors*). If the gentleman faces his own partner and' join
r. hands the same will result, but with l. hands joined, both
left feet will be dedans and r. feet, dehors. Standing side
by side, gentleman's r. and lady's l. will be dedans, the others
are dehors.

Pied Fermé (PEE-AY FER-MAY). Firm foot or shut foot. When the
feet are apart then one is brought tightly to the other.
Example:—Glisser l.f. forward, " fermer " the r.f. that is
close, r.f. to l.f. in 1st, 3rd, or 5th positions.

Pieds ouverts (PEE-AY ZOO-VAIR). Feet opened. The opposite of pied
fermé.

Pigeon, ailes de. (*See* Ailes de pigeon).

Piqué (pas), (PEE-KAY) de la pointe et du talon. Toe and heel points.
(*See* Pointé).

Pirouette (PE-ROO-ET). From low Latin gyruetta, a turn. The performance of one or more complete turns on the toe or ball
of one foot. Some authors assert that at least three such turns
must be made for a pirouette which is exclusively a movement
in theatrical dancing. According to Despreaux this step was
brought from Stuttgart in 1766 by two dancers, Mdlle. Heinel
and Mons. Ferville, who made their debut in the Paris Opera
and astonished the spectators with their pirouettes which were
then unknown. Gardel and Vestris improved on them. Great
suppleness is required for their easy execution. They may be
made à plat (on the flat), or pointé (on the tips), with or without movements of the arms. Many theories have been given for
the execution of this step, but that of Blasis is the best. He
says : " A pirouette of three or four turns in the second position, and stopped in the same, or in an attitude offers the
greatest proof of a dancer's uprightness. Nothing is more
difficult in dancing than the performance of this pirouette.
He whom nature hath favoured with pliancy and agility is
always able to perform them gracefully. Let your body be
steadily fixed on your legs before you begin your pirouettes,
and place your arms in such a position as to give additional
force to the impulse that sends you round, as also to act as a
balance to counterpoise every part of your body as it revolves
on your toes." The different pirouettes are : *pirouettes à petits
battemens* on the instep; *à rond de jambe*; *avec fouetté*; *en
attitude*; *en arabesque*; *sur le cou-de-pied*; en dedans à la
seconde; pirouette renversée; pirouette composeés, etc."
With regard to the theory given, it is based upon principles
which are geometrically demonstrated; their variety is great,
but all requre the greatest attention in correctly possessing
and keeping the centre of gravity. This centre, being the
resultant of all the forces of the body, assures the dancer his
solidity, so long as he is able to practice the elementary principles which have been given to him.

Pirouette simple. On the "demi pointé": "plier" (bend) the knees "degager" a foot to the second position (these two movements are called "preparation to the pirouette") bring back this foot by crossing it in front of the other leg, and turn "en avant" or "en arrière" on the foot which is on the ground. One must "epauler" (lean the shoulder) strongly towards the side one wishes to turn, that is to say in advancing or in receding the shoulder in the direction taken by the turning foot. To terminate, assemblé "devant" or "derrière" the foot which is lifted.

The pirouette is called "ouverte" (opened) when the body turns "en avant," and "fermée" (closed) when the body turns "en arrière."

Pirouette a la seconde position, or **grande pirouette.** Plier the knees and lift up a leg rapidly to the height of the hip, and turn "en avant" or "en arrière" on the tip of the other foot in maintaining stretched out the lifted leg. The part of the shoulder is still more important in this pirouette than in the preceding, and must remain perpendicular with the hip.

Pirouette with attitude, or **arabesque.** The pirouette is thus called when, after the grande pirouette, the dancer lets his lifted leg fall back in order to place himself "en attitude" or "en arabesque." This pirouette is similar to the "point d'orgue" in music.

Pirouettes with **ronds de jambe,** or **petits battements sur le coude-pied.** The lifted leg describes some precipitated ronds de jambe en l'air, or some petits battements while the body turns on the other; this last pirouette always produces much effect in theatrical dance. Vestris executed them with such perfection that he represented the rays of the sun in producing them in his "grands ballets."

Pirouettes-*execution.* When *en dehors* (outward) commence in 3rd position, and is done in three temps but continuously connected without interruption. Assuming the pirouette to be on l.f., the r.f. must be in forward 3rd position, then (1) Elevé (rise) on l. ball simultaneously raising r.f. in 2nd elevation and both arms to height of shoulders. (2) Lower the body on both feet in the 2nd plié (bended position), by which the right side is carried obliquely forward by an outward turning of the l.f. on the point, simultaneously carry r. arm round to front somewhat lower. (3) Quickly raise r.f. from floor and rising on the l. point, turn quickly assisted by the swing of the arms.

Pirouettes en l'air are turns of the entire body with both feet off the floor. These turns are sometimes called "*volta*" or "*rivolta.*"

Pistolets. (*See* Ailes de Pigeon).

Pivoter (PIV-OT-AY). To pivot on one or both feet.

Plier, Plié (PLEE-AY). Flexion or *bending* of one or both knees in preparation for any step.

Point. Any movement made with the toe pointing to the ground; when made with the heel it is known as *piqué* (*see* next article),

Pointé du talon or **Piqué** (PEE-KAY). Movements made with the point of the heel, toe pointing upwards, as in toe-and-heel of the hornpipe.

Polka. Originally a war dance. " Polk " or " pulk " is the name of a regiment of Cossacks, and is an old Scythian word originally applied to a tribe. It therefore included both the male and female members of a nomadic horde. This derivation accounts, therefore, for those remarkable features which distinguish it from every other dance. The spurs, the tapping of the ground with the heel, flourishing a battle-axe in the air and other gestures of a warlike nature, are all the accompaniments of the polka when danced by the Servians, among whom it was first observed. Another account gives the inventor of the dance as Anna Stezak, a farm servant at Elbsteinitz, near Prague, about 1830. The room in which she was accustomed to dance being of small dimensions, the movements of her feet were short, and so the dance was called the " Pulka " dance, that is, the " half " dance. The music according to this account was written down by a local musician named Neruda. Yet another account claims that the dance was invented in 1834 by a native of Moksic, in Bohemia.

It is a round dance for two persons. Position as for the waltz. Gentleman's step—count (*and*) a preliminary hop on r.f. (1) Glissade l.f. to 2nd position. (2) Coupé en avant r.f. against l.f. turning a quarter-circle. (3) Coupé en arrière l.f. against r.f., turning another quarter-circle, thus the three temps will complete half-circle; repeat with other foot (count *and*, 1, 2, 3.) Ladies do the counterpart.

Polka Mazurka. (See Mazurka).

Polonaise. A promenade with which public and private dances were opened. It consisted of various figures.

Port des Bras. (PORT DAY BRAH). (*See* Bras).

Porter (PAW-TAY). To carry the foot, that is when it is not glided.

Positions. (*See* A.B.C.)

Poule, la. (*See* Quadrilles).

Poursuite, la (POOR-SWEET). The pursuit. A couple dancing straightforward as a variation in a round dance, instead of turning. As a rule, the gentleman should go backward.

Poussé (*poo-say*). Sometimes as in the Mazurka, there is a strongly felt knock of the feet, this is a coupé poussé.

Prelude. The opening eight bars of music preceding the 2nd, 3rd, 4th and 5th figures of square dances. The opening eight bars of the 1st figure is called " introduction."

Promenade (PROM-ENAHD). An ordinary walking step in strict musical tempo. *Grande Promenade,* the couples walk completely round the circle; *Demi-Promenade,* half-round.

Pyrrhic (PIR-RIK). Grecian warlike dances. So called either through Phrrhus, son of Achilles, who, it is reported, performed them first at his father's funeral, or, through Pyrrhicus the Spartan, who is said to have invented them. The dancers were fully armed.

Q

Quadrille. Originally it was called *Contredanse,* an English country dance. Since 1710 introduced in France it consists of several figures generally performed by four couples placed in the form of a square. In all such squares dances, the couples standing with their backs to the music are the *first couples,* the *second couples* face the first couples; the third couples are on the right of the first; the *fourth couples* face the third. Originally, there were six figures. At Almack's Rooms, the Quadrille known as Hart's " First Set " consisted of Pantalon, l'Été, La Poule, Trenise, Pastorale, Finale. There were many " sets " arranged by Hart (I have 35 such sets). Weippert also arranged 31 " sets." The music is written partly in 6-8 tempo (M.M. 88 = ♪'), partly 2-4 (M.M. 84=♪). Usually the first figure commences in 6-8 tempo, the second figure in 2-4 tempo. It is as well to mention that the first eight bars are played only as an introduction to which the dancers have but to listen in order to commence the dancing of the figure in punctual time.

(The opinion that the introduction is only to give time to the couples to bow to each other as well to the corner is an erroneous one. The object of the introduction is to inform the dancers of the change of tempo and give them the opportunity to commence in that tempo. To make a bow or curtsey twelve times in one quadrille is as useless as it is in bad taste. One curtsey at the commencement of the first figure and two curtseys at the end, meet all the requirements).

This explains the reason why the first eight bars of the music of each figure is also its closing part. Further, it is well to mention that the music of the first figure, Pantalon, must be played twice, all the others four times.

In recent times artistic steps are seldom seen in Quadrilles, on the other hand inartistic and single steps are frequently used. The correctness of this observation is undeniable. The neglect of artistic steps may be attributed to indolence and love of ease, especially with ladies who desire to preserve their toilettes. Society has voluntarily relinquished shining through the ability of the feet; but they have in no way banished grace from the various movements of the body on the contrary, they have known how to preserve it in employing the simple dancing steps in a gracefully gliding manner. This natural gliding of the foot, accompanied by an expression of ease which seems to indicate artistic steps, only in the slightest form, in no way excludes a previous knowledge of them, and is not easily imitated by those who have not the advantage of previous thorough tuition. To oppose the prevalent fashion would be a doubtful and very rash undertaking.

EXPLANATION OF THE QUADRILLE FIGURES MOST IN USE.

1. LE PANTALON. 8 *bars* . . . . CHAINE ANGLAISE ENTIÉRE.—Two couples standing opposite each other have for their object the change of places. They advance and present the right hand to the vis-a-vis, then in the second movement the left hand to partners, thus by a *demi-chaine anglaise* they reach the opposite side. This repeated (a second half of the *chaine anglaise*) they regain their former places. In modern times the same movement is made but the giving of hands is omitted and is called " Right and Left."

4 *bars* . . . . BALANCÉ.—Now called "Setting to partners." Each couple facing partners and

4 *bars* . . . . UN TOUR DE (*deux*) MAINS—they give both hands to execute one *tour* to the right in place.

If only one hand, say the right, is given, the tour must be made in the contrary direction, also if no hand is given.

8 *bars* . . . . CHAINE DES DAMES.—Both opposite ladies in changing places give the right hand when they meet and then the left hand to the opposite gentleman. The gentlemen, when their partners leave their places, advance sideways to the right to meet the opposite lady with the left hand. Both couples repeat these movements.

4 *bars* . . . . DEMI-PROMENADE.—(The expression *Demi queue du chat* is out of date). At the end of the last figure each gentleman held partner's left hand. They now cross the right hands over the left and both couples change places, the gentleman passing left shoulder to left shoulder and the ladies describe the outer circle to the opposite side.

4 *bars* . . . . DEMI-CHAINE ANGLAISE.—With this the couples return to their places.

The other two couples repeat these movements.

2. L'ÉTÉ. 4 *bars* . . . . EN AVANT DEUX (ET EN ARRIÈRE). One gentleman and opposite lady advance and retire.

4 *bars* . . . . A DROITE ET À GAUCHE.—They move sideways to the right and to the left.

4 *bars* . . . . TRAVERSÉ.—They change places right shoulder to right shoulder.

127

4 *bars* . . . . A DROITE ET À GAUCHE.—They move again sideways to the right and to the left.

4 *bars* . . . . RETRAVERSÉ ET BALANCÉ —They return in the same way to their places and are received by their partners (who simultaneously with the retraversé did the balancé) and

4 *bars* . . . . UN TOUR DE (*deux*) MAINS, each couple is reunited. (This is repeated three times for the other couples).

This figure as described, is the " Single Été." The modern figure is the " Double Été" and is done thus:—1st and 2nd couples advance and retire, cross over, advance and retire, recross, set to partners and turn.

3. LA POULE, (Sometimes the sequence of figures is altered and the *Pastourelle* is the third, *Poule* the fourth and *Trénis* the fifth figures. Strictly, the *Pastourelle* and *Trénis* should never be danced in a Quadrille but only one of them. If, however, both figures are required in one Quadrille it would be advisable to place *Poule* between them because *Pastourelle* and *Trénis* resemble each other somewhat).

4 *bars* . . . . TRAVERSÉ.—A gentleman and opposite lady change places passing right shoulder to right shoulder.

4 *bars* . . . . RE-TRAVERSÉ PAR LA MAIN GAUCHE.—Both return presenting left hands joined and the right hands to their partners to perform,

4 *bars* . . . . BALANCÉ QUATRE EN LIGNE.—Balancé four in a line.

4 *bars* . . . . DEMI-PROMENADE.—Both couples change their places, the gentlemen leading passing left shoulder to left shoulder.

4 *bars* . . . . EN AVANT DEUX ET EN ARRIÈRE.—The gentleman and lady dancing the figure advance and retire.

4 *bars* . . . . DOS À DOS.—(Recently a tour de mains came into use). Moving round each other right shoulder to right shoulder and back to back, they return to the places from which they started.

Nowadays, the pair advance and retire, advance again with reverence and retire.

4 *bars* . . . . EN AVANT QUATRE ET EN ARRIÈRE.—Both couples advance and retire.

4 *bars* . . . . DEMI-CHAINE ANGLAISE.—Regain original positions with this.

Repeated three times for the other dancers.

4. LA PASTOURELLE. 8 *bars* . . . . UN CAVALIER ET SA DAME EN AVANT ET EN ARRIÈRE DEUX FOIS.—One couple advance and retire, advance once more, the gentleman retires alone while the lady crosses to the left of the opposite gentleman who has meanwhile taken his partner's left hand thus preparing to receive the opposite lady with his left hand.

8 bars . . . . EN AVANT TROIS DEUX FOIS.—The three advance and retire, twice.

8 bars . . . . LE CAVALIER SEUL.—The single gentleman dances a solo on a self-chosen line gradually approaching his partner.

This is now altered to:—the set of three advance again, the gentleman leaving the ladies with opposite gentleman and retire alone. Set of three advance and retire, all advance and form a circle.

4 bars . . . . DEMI TOUR DE ROND À GAUCHE—Both gentlemen take their partners' left hands with their right and move sideways in a circle to the left (for the purpose of changing places, to accomplish which they part in the rond) and take the places of the opposite couple and

4 bars . . . . DEMI-CHAINE ANGLAISE by which they regain their original places.

Three repetitions for the three other couples.

5. LA TRÉNIS   (*Named after its inventor, Trénitz, who in his time*—1800—*was a famous dancer*).

8 bars . . . . UN CAVALIER ET SA DAME EN AVANT ET EN ARRIÈRE DEUX FOIS.—Exactly like the first figure of the *Pastourelle.*

8 bars . . . . LE CAVALIER TRAVERSÉ AU MILIEU DE DEUX DAMES.—The single gentleman advances to the opposite one, the movement ending in a demi-tour (half-turn) whilst both ladies move in a circle twice round him and facing him. This circling ends by the ladies returning to places.

4 bars . . . . BALANCÉ.—As in *Pantalon.*

4 bars . . . . TOUR DE (deux)MAINS.—As in *Pantalon.*

Repeated three times for the other couples.

Modern:—Grand circle. All advance and retire. Turn partners. Repeat second figure. Repeat three times.

Another variation known as " Flirtation " Figure. Grand circle advance and retire. All set to and turn corners. Promenade round sixteen steps. Repeat three times.

6. LA FINALE.   *4 bars* . . . . CHASSÉ CROISÉ HUIT· All the ladies move sideways to the left and, simultaneously, the gentlemen move in a line crossing sideways behind their partners to the right adding a demi-balancé which is to be executed facing each other and must be looked upon as a leave-taking.

4 bars . . . . DE-CHASSÉ HUIT.—In the same manner return to places.

4 bars . . . . MOULINET DES DAMES.—All ladies join hands to form a moving star which formation after one tour (circle round) must be maintained until

4 bars . . . . DEMI-BALANCÉ EN MOULINET ET DEMI TOUR DE MAINS, the gentlemen with the left hand take the ladies' left hands thus joining the ladies' star. All perform the *demi-balancé* and the ladies (releasing the right hands and disjointing the star) withdraw from the centre by half a tour de main with the left hand, whilst the gentlemen reach the centre by the same tour de main.

8 *bars* . . . . GRANDE PROMENADE.—Gentlemen with right hand take their partners' right, and the couples following each other, move forward describing a large circle until they reach their original places.

24 *bars* {
EN AVANT DEUX ET EN ARRIÈRE
À DROITE ET À GAUCHE
TRAVERSÉ
À DROITE ET À GAUCHE
RETRAVERSÉ ET BALANCÉ
UN TOUR DE (DEUX) MAINS
} As in the second figure L'Été.

After the *Finale* has been danced four times and *l'été* has also been danced four times, then follows the CODA 24 bars ; CHASSÉ CROISÉ HUIT, MOULINET DES DAMES, DEMI-BALANCÉ ET DEMI-TOUR DE MAINS, and conclude with GRANDE PROMENADE.

Quatre (KAHTR). *See* Entrechat.

Queue de Chat (KER–DER–SHAH). *See* Demi-Promenade, Quadrille figure I.

R

Ramassé (RAH-MAH–SAY).—To pick up. In many dances, such as Spanish, a strong bend of the body occurs combined with a lowering of the arms as if to pick something up from the floor.

Rebours (RE-BOOR, or à l'envers.)—Reverse, as valse à rebours (waltz reverse).

Rebroussale (RE-BROO–SAL.)—The heel position of the foot. (*See* A.B.C. direction).

Redowa.—Round dance in 3-4 tempo. Obsolete. Position as for waltz. *Gentleman's step.*—(1) Glide l.f. to 2nd, (2) glide r.f. to rear of l.f., slightly raising the l.f. (3) drop on l.f. with r.f. up rear. During this the dancers make one-half circle; repeat with r.f. to complete the circle.

Redowaczka.—The Redowa in 2-4 tempo.

Redresser (RE-DRESSAY.)—*See* Allonger.

Reels (Scotch and Irish).—Native dances of these countries. Many descriptive works exist.

Relevé (REL-AVAY).—Relifting or straightening of the knee.

Retombé (RE-TOMBAY).—After a jump (*sauté*) one must perforce come down again on the feet, this is *retombé*. Hence the term used is always *sauté et retombé* (jump and fall again).

Retreversé (RET-REE.VAIR-SAY).—To retraverse, that is to go over the same road. In square dances *traversé* is to cross from one side to the other, *retraversé* is to re-cross, back to places. (See Quadrille fig. 2.)

Révérence. (RAY-VAY-RAHNS).—The lady's curtsey and gentleman's bow.

Reye.—Supposed to be the "Hay" of Chaucer's time, about 1340 (*See* Solomon's Jig).

Rhythm.—The time or beat of the music with which the dance must be in strict accord.

Rigaudon (RIG-O-DAW.)—Derives its name from Regaudon, a dancing-master of Marseilles, who brought it from Provence (1485.) The French Revolution killed it. The music in common time consists of two parts of eight bars each. Singing accompanied the music, the words beginning "Ah, Chloe, when I prove my passion," (date 1709) is a good one. Each figure takes eight bars. Both dancers stand side by side but do not hold hands. (1) Glide and make four running steps, turn and pose; repeat opposite foot. (2) Turn to left and right alternately four times going backward. (3) To the right diagonally with running steps, turn and pose; repeat to left. (4) Two hops and turn, repeat, run diagonally to right and turn, same to left, arms straight out. (5) Half turn to left, same to right, whole turn to left, repeat. (6) Arms above head, three steps to l., turn to l., repeat to r., hop round and pose r. hand down l. hand overhead. (7) Balancez four times on l.f., same on r. f. and pose. The head and arm movements are important.

Regaudon, *pas.*—Jeté followed by fouetté.

Ritournelle (RITOOR-NEL).—A flourish. Before arranging a square dance it is customary for the orchestra to play eight or sixteen bars of the first figure, this is *ritournelle*, or signal to the dancers to enter the ballroom and arrange themselves in their sets for the dance.

Rivolta or **Volta.**—A pirouette en l'air (*See* Pirouette).

Rond. Any movement in a circle.—*Grand Ronde*, a grand circle.

Rond de **Bras** (RAWN-DER-BRAH).—Rounding the arms.

Rond de **Jambe** (RAWN-DER-JHAHM).—Rounding the leg in a circle either en dedans or en dehors (inward or outward) en terre or en l'air (on the floor or raised.)

Ruement, Ruer, (RU-MAHN, RU-AY).—A kick, to kick. Forcibly throwing the leg into an open position, as though kicking.

Russe *pas.*—(*See* Basque).

S

Saraband.—The word, derived from the Arabic, means "noise." The dance came from Spain about the twelfth century and in olden times was danced in groups to the sound of bells and castagnets. Rather wild in its character in those days it was danced only by women, but passing into France it naturally became beautified and greatly influenced France when it led European dancing. When seventy years of age Arbeau gives a description in " L'Orchesographie." Under Louis the Melancholy (Louis XIII) the dance became fashionable as a solo for man or woman. Music is in ¾ tempo, is in two parts of eight bars each. Each figure occupies eight bars. (1) Raise r.f. and step forward, turn to right and pose, repeat with l.f., again with r.f. (2) Pas bourrée r.f., same l.f., again r.f., turn to the right then to the left. (3) Change the foot going to the left with the Spanish hip movement (pas glissé) twice; coupé and pose with movements of the head going to right and left with the music; repeat all to right. (4) Spring on l.f., stretch r. leg to rear and bow. Repeat with r.f. turning to right and posing. Repeat the whole, then raise r.f. and step forward, same l.f., same r.f., point l.f. and pose. Repeat the whole and end with curtsey.

Sauté, Sauter (so-TAY).—Jump or hop, the same term applies to both.

Scalp Dance.—Of the Sioux, Apaches and Cheyennes. Its title describes the dance.

Schottische or **Schottisch.**—In Bavaria, in 1844, there was danced a round dance called " Rhinelander." The music was in 2-4 but played so slowly as to resemble common time. In France, England and Russia it was called " Scottish." The application of this name to the dance is impossible to explain, but it was afterwards called " Scottish Waltz." It is now played in common time, the complete movement occupying four bars or 16 counts. *Gentleman's step—waltz position.*—(1) Glide l.f. to 2nd pos. (2) close r.f. to 3rd rear (3) l.f. to 2nd pos. (4) hop on l.f. with r.f. raised rear of l.f. (1 bar.) Reverse, moving to the right (1 bar), (1) glide l.f. to 2nd, (2) hop, (3, 4) repeat with r.f. (1 bar), repeat last bar (1 bar); during the last two bars a complete circle or two circle should be made. Often the last two bars are waltzed, making a complete waltz movement to each bar.

Scissor-Step.—(*See* Sissonne).

Scopia.—Ancient Greek dance in which the dancers held their hands, funnel shaped, to the eyes as though the better to see distant objects.

Seguidillas.—Dancing plays an important part in Spanish national life. The Bolero is an important dance and *Seguidillas* means a *continuation*; the music for both dances is the same continued by the voice. When the Boleros are sung to a guitar and castagnette accompaniment they are called *Seguidillas Boleras.* Then there is the *Seguidillas Manchegas* for four, six or eight persons; this is sprightly in its movements and a great favourite with the lower orders. The *Seguidillas Taleadas* is a mixture of Cachucha and Bolero. Music 3-4 tempo. The dancers, are placed in two lines facing each other, then they pass across to opposite side, recross, parade and promenade. All the Boleros originally consisted of five parts, (1) *the paseo* or promenade which served as an introduction, (2) *traversias* or crossing which is done before and after the *differencias* (3) when a change of steps takes place followed by (4) *finales* and (5) *bien parado,* a graceful attitude or grouping.

Siciliano.—A graceful pastoral dance of Sicily. Music by flageolet and tambourine in 6-4, 6-8 time. It figures at many weddings and festivities. In Sicily, the man chooses his partner and they dance together holding a hankerchief then he retires. After dancing a short solo, she chooses another partner and so the dance continues. Suitable music, Purcell's Suite No. 11. The dance—(1) Step forward r.f., then l.f. and turn. Step to left, step to right and turn. Repeat the whole with tambourine accompaniment. (2) Pirouette to i., point r.f.; repeat and chassé forward (this occupies 7 bars) point l.f. and pose arms raised playing the tambourine for eighth bars. (3) Four pas de basques forward and four back, then pirouette to right, four pas de basques forward, pirouette to left and four back. (4) Point l. toe four times, then back with r.f. and pirouette to right; repeat other foot. (5) Eight pas de basques forward, turning on the fifth, sixth, seventh and eighth.

Sir Roger de Coverley.—Old English country dance. This was usually the final dance of the evening and is still in vogue at Christmas in the good old English country houses and causes great hilarity. The dancers are arranged in two lines, gentlemen on one side, ladies on the other side. (Fig. 1) The top lady and bottom gentleman advance to the centre of the lines give right hands, swing round and retire to places. Bottom lady and top gentleman repeat. (Fig. 2) repeat with l. hand. (Fig. 3) repeat with both hands. (Fig. 4) top lady and bottom gentleman advance to centre and pass round each other *dos-a-dos* (back to back) and retire to places. Bottom lady and top gentleman repeat. (Fig. 5) This figure is seldom done although it is very effective. The top lady crosses round second gentleman then between second and third ladies, then between third and fourth gentlemen, then between fourth and fifth ladies and continue the serpentine movement to the end of the line. The top gentleman does the same simultaneously commencing to pass round the second lady then between second and third gentleman and so on until they meet at the same moment at the bottom of the lines. (Fig. 6) the couple joining inside hands run down the centre of the line to their places. (Fig. 7) the same couple again run down the centre to the bottom and raise both hands high, simultaneously all the other dancers make a quarter-turn facing the top. The couple who will now be top turn outward and, all the others following, run to the bottom of the room, take partner's hand and passing under the upraised arms run to the top, all the others following. Couple No. 2 will now be No. 1 and so on, the previous top couple being now at the bottom. Repeat from fig. 1., ad lib.

Sissonne (SIS-SONN).—(*See* Ciseaux).

Soubresaut (SOO-BR-SO). - A sudden leap or start. Glide one foot forward to the rear or to the side, raise the other in any direction and jump on the foot which is on the ground. It is a jump executed on one foot or hopping.

Soutenu (SOO-TER-NOO).—Supported or sustained. The stepping foot which receives the weight of the body is followed by the other stretched foot in a dragging manner and remains in the first, or moving sideways to the second position in the air, to procede then to the second step when the other foot goes through the same dragging process.

Space.—In a ballroom, each couple should have 4 feet of the length and 4 feet of the breadth. In a hall 36 by 24, accommodation is provided for seating, 9 couples on each long side and 6 couples on each broad side or 30 couples in all. More than these will crowd the hall. Twenty couples would require a hall of 384 square feet, say 24 by 16 or its equivalent, etc.

Stage-Dancing.- (*See* Theatre).

Sun-dance.—On the occasion of a young Sioux Indian being admitted into the ranks of the braves, this dance is executed, during which the newcomer undergoes the most frightful tortures, in order to test his efficiency as a warrior.

Sword-dances.—Of Scotland and Northern England. Dances performed on crossed swords. For full descriptions see " Sword Dances " published by Novello & Co., London.

T

Tacqueté or **Taqueté** (TAHK-ETA). To stamp on the points of the foot. The arms for this should be in 1st position.

Talonné (TAHL-LONAY).—Tap one heel against the other without displacing the soles which should serve as pivots for turning the feet in and out.

Tambourin.—Many dances of Southern Europe and Central America are accompanied by the dancer's beat of this instrument.

Tango or **El Tango** (TAHN-GO)—This dance was originally Cuban, whence it passed to Spain then to the Argentine Republic, where it became the popular dance of the Gauchos (*cow boys*), who danced it in couples with a virility and realism which are the real features of the steps. Imported a short while ago into Paris by a few young Argentines its licentious character pleased the tastes of the habitués of the cafés of Montmatre. The French dancing Masters modified it so that it should conform more with our ideas, and with fixed rules and a regulated type of music, the Tango became popular with a world-wide reputation. The Spanish and Argentine Tango have nothing in common with the Parisian Tango, only the music presents certain analogies which is natural, as the dances have a common origin. The dance and music combined are very alluring and merit the closest attention. At the first accents of the orchestra, all lassitude disappears, new life seems to circulate within the dancers, new ardour seems to give them the zest of new youth. It is an exquisite movement which pleases the eye and enchants the spirit and senses, and the dancers for the time dwell in the domain of dreams.

The Tango Argentine is composed of twelve steps: (1) EL PASEO (*la promenade*); (2) EL MARCHA (*la marche*); (3) EL MEDIO CORTE (*le demi coupé*); (4) EL CORTE (*le coupé*); (5) LA MEDIA LUNA (*la demi lune*); (6) EL CHASE (*les chasses*); (7) EL CRUZADO (*les croisés*); (8) EL OCHO ARGENTINO (*le huit argentin*); (9) EL RUEDA (*la roue*); (10) EL FROTTADO (*le frotté*); (11) EL ABANICO (*l'eventail*); (12) EL MOLINETTE (*le moulinet*). These steps require precise explanations for the pupil to dance, the Tango cannot, therefore, be learnt from any printed description, but must be studied under a properly qualified teacher.

Taper (TAH-PAY).—To put down the foot with energy. Stamping.

Tarentellé.– National Neapolitan dance ; the name is attributed to the spider tarantula, the only cure for whose poisonous bite was to dance and dance until the poison was eliminated.

Ta-Tao (TAH-TAH-O).—(*See* separate sheet).

Tempête la. An obsolete country dance. Was danced in lines of four facing each other.

Tempo (TAHM-PO). The musical time occupied by each step. Also, the counting of the beats in each bar of music, as 2-4 tempo (two in the bar), 3-4 tempo (three in the bar), 6-8 tempo (six in the bar), common or 4-4 tempo (four to the bar). Also the length of time occupied by each beat, this is usually written as so many beats of crochets, quavers or minims as played per minute and timed by a pendulum attached to clockwork, known as Maeltzel's Metronome, and written M.M. 50, M.M. 60, M.M. 70, as the case may be, meaning 50, 60 or 70 beats per minute. The following tempo table should be studied:—WALTZ ♩ M.M. 72 ; Galop ♩ M.M. 76 ; Polka ♩ M.M. 104 ; Redowa ♩ M.M. 60 ; Schottische ♩ M.M. 76 ; Mazurka M.M. 56 ; Quadrille ♩ M.M. 104 ; Lancers ♩ M.M. 104 ; Varsovienne ♩ M.M. 54 ; Court Quadrille ♩ MM. 76.

Temps (TAHM).—A syllable or part of a step. Example—a *pas* de basque consists of three *temps*.

135

Tendre (TAHNDR).—To stretch. The opposite of plié.

Tendu pas (PAH TAHNDOO) or **Zephyr**).—A stretched step. Example—stand r.f. raised to 4th forward elevation. (1) r.f. coupé dessus, making l.f. come to 4th rear. (2) hop on r.f. during which the stretched l.f. goes to the forward 4th elevation lightly touching the floor when passing r.f.

Terre-à-terre (TEHR-AH-TEHR).—A gliding style of dancing, with small steps connected with each other lightly gliding on the floor, in contrast to the lifting of the foot (en l'air). In ballroom dancing steps terre-à-terre are decidedly in greater use.

Tetara.—Greek tragic dance by four persons with legs and arms entwining in cadence.

Theatre.—The basis of modern threatrical dancing undoubtedly owes its origin to the labours of l'Academie Nationale de Danse de Paris, founded by Louis XIV in 1661. (*For the names of the Academicians see* " *Academy* "). A good teacher of theatrical dancing should have an intimate knowledge of the preparation for and construction of ballets and of the plastic art; he should be prepared to illustrate every step employed in the dance; he should be a master of music; he should have control of language; he should be acquainted with the history, costume and lives of all peoples; he should possess imagination, inspiration, judgment, a good memory, inexhaustible patience and perfect taste. All these qualities, and a few others, are indispensable for a teacher of ballet.

Theatrical dancing is a very difficult art acquired only after long and arduous study and practice under the direction of a capable teacher. Those pirouetts and other movements which charm us have cost the dancer many weary years of incessant labour. Unless the pupil is prepared to persevere and surmount all obstacles little or no progress can be made. The teacher must constantly give words of encouragement. Seven or eight years of age is not too young to commence instruction, the limbs are then pliable and may be moulded for dancing purposes.

Terms most in use during the lesson:—

ABAISSER
AILES DE PIGEON
ASSEMBLÉ
ATTITUDE
BAISSER
BALANCÉ
BALLONNÉ
BALLOTTÉS
BASQUE (pas de)
BATTEMENTS (grands and petits)
BATTRE
BATTU
BOURRÉE
BOURRÉE (pas de)

GLISSÉ
HOLUBIEC
JETÉ ASSEMBLÉ
JETÉ EN TOURNANT
JETÉ (pas)
JETÉ RELEVÉ
LEVÉ (pas or temps)
MARCHÉ (ordinaire or militaire)
OPPOSITION
PAS COURUS
PAS SUR LES POINTES
PIEDS (fermé, ouvert, en dedans or en dehors)
PIROUETTE

BERCEAU
BRISÉ dessus, dessous
BRAS (5 positions)
BRISÉ, DESSUS, DESSOUS
CABRIOLE
CHANGEMENT DE JAMBE
CHANGEMENT DE PIED
CHANGEMENT DE TALON
CHASSÉS
CISEAUX
CONTRETEMPS
COUPÉ, dessus, dessous, demi-coupé
DÉBOÎTÉ
DÉGAGÉ
DÉTOURNÉ OR DÉROULÉ
DÉVELLOPPÉ
ECART EN L'AIR OR À TERRE
ECARTÉ (temps)
ECHAPPÉ (temps)
ELEVÉ, MARCHÉ
ELEVER on 1 or 2 feet
ELEVÉS (pas)
ELEVATIONS
EMBOITÉS
EN HAUT
EN L'AIR
EN TERRE
EN TOURNANT
ENTRECHAT
ÉPAULEMENT
FLEURET
FOUETTÉ
FRAPPÉ
FROTTÉ
GARGOUILLADE
GLISSADE

PLIÉ
PORT DES BRAS
PORTER
POSITION (1st, 2nd, 3rd, 4th, 5th)
RAMASSÉ
RELEVÉ
REPEAT
RHYTHM
RIGODON or SISSONNE DOUBLE
ROND DE JAMBE (dessus, dessous, etc).
SAUT DE CHAT, BOND
SISSONNE DÉTOURNÉ
SISSONNE RELEVÉ (pas)
SISSONNE (temps)
SOUBRESAUT
SOULEVÉ
TACQUETÉ
TAPER
TEMPS DE CUISSE
TEMPS DE L'ANGE or PLANER
TENDRE
TENDU (pas)
TERRE-À-TERRE
TÊTE (the head, 5 positions, i.e., right, left, forward, backward and fixed).
TIRÉ
TOMBÉ
TORTILLER
TOUR EN L'AIR
TOURNER
TRIOLET
TROT DE CHEVAL
ZÉPHYR (pas de)

The daily practice at first should not exceed one-and-a-half hours.

1st. Twenty minutes' bar practice. The opening and bending of the feet and legs in all positions on the ground and in the air.

2nd. Thirty minutes to exercises in adage, aplomb, and pirouettes of every description.

3rd. Twenty minutes to changements de pieds, practice on the points and the various battement steps.

4th. Twenty minutes to enchaînements.

In all dancing schools there should be on the walls pictures or blackboards on which are represented positions of the body, of the legs and arms in opposition, of certain geometrical lines, of perpendiculars, horizontals, obliques, right angles, obtuse angles and acute angles.

The teacher must demonstrate each step for the imitation of the pupil, who must endeavour to make a faithful reproduction of the teacher's movements. Care must be taken not to over-fatigue the pupil who occasionally needs rest as well as the teacher.

In the class room, there should be what is called a " bar.' This is a round pole (which can be easily grasped) placed horizontally round the room, at a height of from 36 to 40 inches from the floor (on supports) and standing about nine to twelve inches from the wall and parallel to it. In all practices, the pupil stands sideways grasping the bar with the right hand for all movements with the left leg and with the left hand for movements with the right leg. Any number of pupils may practice simultaneously by facing in the same direction. The exercises of the legs, arms and body should never be interrupted; the dancer who misses the exercises for a day cannot recover what has been lost, and he will lose some of the force and agility acquired after so much labour. In the exercises, the pupil must work with both legs alike that they may get equal force, taking care of the carriage of the body and the arms in the attitudes and arabesques making them with perfect aplomb, equilibrium and grace. He must become vigourous without angularity, rigidity or stiffness, that the cuts and crossings of the entrechat may be clean and sharply defined. He must acquire a light, easy aerial elevation, lightly skimming the ground as though the feet are tenderly kissing it.

The student must first be well grounded in the five positions of the feet and arms (with their variations) after which the exercises may be proceeded with. Repeat all the exercises several times, then the same with the other foot.

POSITIONS DES BRAS (positions of the arms) as taught at the "Paris Opéra School."

1st *Position.*—The two hands forward with arms rounded at the height of the waist. (Fig. 5, but slightly higher).

2nd *Position.*—The arms outstretched horizontally at the side at the height of the shoulder, parallel to the feet which should also be in the 2nd position (Fig. 1.)

3rd *Position.*—The r. arm half-rounded (*demi-arondi*) at the height of the waist (1st pos.); the l. arm in an attitude forming a half-circle over the head (Fig. 7) (*demi-couronne*). The arms change their positions when l.f. is placed before r.f.

4th *Position.*—En demi-bras.—The two arms rounded in front of the body, the elbows elevated, the fingers almost touching at the height of the pit of the stomach. This position is generally employed for the commencing and finishing a variation.

5th *Position.*—The two arms are aloft, the elbows rounded elevated, the palms down and fingers grouped—the palm should be turned inward, that is, the back of the hand is towards the ceiling, the arms forming a *couronne* (*crown*) (fig. 7). This pose assumes the form of a lyre and is known as the "*lyre pose.*"

DERIVATIVE POSITIONS OF THE ARMS.

1st Position.—En opposition.—One arm is put forward outstretched the other the same to the rear. In this position equally one arm may be held aloft while the other is directed to the ground.

2nd Position.—Double bras.—One arm across the chest, the hand carried at the height of the shoulder—the left shoulder for the right arm and vice-versa, the other arm a little higher than the 2nd elementary position, the palms of both hands directed to the same side.

3rd Position.—Bras convexes.—One arm in the 4th elementary position and the other in demi-couronne (Fig. 7).

4th Position.—One arm in 4th, the other in 2nd elementary positions.

THE HAND should always be held classically, the fingers grouped so that the thumb touches the points of the two middle fingers very lightly, the little finger hanging loosely, the forefinger pointing slightly forward: all naturally, without force.

POSITIONS OF THE BODY AND HEAD.

1st Position.—The body or head is normal.

2nd Position.—The body or head inclined to one side or of one to the other.

3rd Position.—The body or head turned to the right or left: this position is called *" epaulé ou de profil."*

4th Position.—The body or head leaning forward.

5th Position.—The body or head backward.

It is indispensable for the pupil to go from any one position to any other without hesitation. Once they are known separately, they can be combined. Example:—Feet and arms, both in 1st pos.; arms and feet in 2nd pos.; 5th of feet, 3rd derivative of arms; 5th of the body and feet and 3rd elementary of arms. Thousands of such combinations can be made and the study of them is very interesting.

Exercise 1. DÉGAGÉ ON THE 5TH TO THE 2ND POSITION. Feet in 5th pos., arms extended sideways level with the shoulder in 2nd pos. Glide the point of r.f. to 2nd pos. the toe down and heel raised without moving the left foot nor moving the arms. Draw r.f. to 5th front, then 2nd, then 5th rear.

Exercise 2. DEMI-ROND DE JAMBE À TERRE FROM 1ST POS. Heels touching in 1st pos., the r. arm in 2nd pos. (fig. 1), l. arm in 4th pos. Glide the point of r.f. to 4th forward, then to the 2nd at the side and continue to 4th rear and finish without pause in 1st pos. *Do not forget to change all arm positions when changing the exercises with the other foot.*

Exercise 3. DÉGAGÉ À LA DEMI-HAUTEUR.—Feet in 1st pos., arm in 2nd pos., other hand grasping bar. Rise on the r. points, the toes only on the floor, heels well raised with the weight on r. toes. Stretch out the raised l. leg to the 2nd pos. at the side, the toe forced pointing downward. On returning the foot, bend the l. knee and pass the heel (toe pointed well-down) close to the r. instep, the l. knee also slightly bent—as in a pirouette—and continue (Fig. IX).

Exercise 4.   ROND DE JAMBE EN L'AIR.—Feet 1st pos., l. arm 2nd pos., grasp bar with r. hand. Rise on r. points, raise l. heel and stretch out the leg well-raised to 4th forward, slowly move it round, still outstretched, to 2nd pos., then, without interruption to 4th rear, thus, the leg at the same height describes a half-circle commencing forward and finishing rear as in exercise 2, and regain 1st pos.

Exercise 5.   PLIÉ IN ALL 5 POSITIONS.—Feet 2nd pos. (fig. 2) arms 2nd pos. (fig. 1). Bend the knees (fig. 8) outward, the body upright. To complete the plié, bend more, so that the thigh will come to the height of the knees. Practice in all positions, with the bar and without.

Exercise 6.   LES POINTES.—Rise on the points in all positions.

Exercise 7.   GRANDS BATTEMENTS.—The feet in 5th, arms in 2nd positions. Raise the left heel, bending the ankle-bone and raise the leg to the height of the other knee, to 2nd elevation (count 1). Bring sharply to 3rd or 5th rear (count 2). Raise leg again (1), bring to 3rd or 5th front (2). Repeat from 4th front elevation and from 4th rear elevation. *Petits battements.*—These are made in exactly the same way but the point of the foot remains on the floor for count 1.

Exercise 8.   DEVELOPPÉS EN ATTITUDES DIFFERENTES (ADAGE).—Feet in 5th, arms in 2nd positions. Slowly raise l. heel and unfold the leg until it is fully stretched out to 2nd elevation level with the knee, or higher; the l. arm goes over the head in a demi-couronne, r. arm remaining in 2nd. Then return the leg to 5th pos.

Exercise 9.   DEVELLOPPÉ TO 4TH POSITION.—The arms rounded over the head (en couronne) the left leg is developed to fourth forward elevation and returned to 5th pos.

Exercise 10.   DEVELLOPPÉ TO 4TH CROSSED.—L. arm demi-couronne, r. arm in 2nd. Develop the r. leg to crossed 4th forward elevation; also 4th rear.

Exercise 11.   FIRST OPEN ATTITUDE IN 4TH REAR OF R. LEG. R. arm en couronne, l. arm in 2nd pos. and the body to the right.

Exercise 12.   SECOND ATTITUDE CROSSED TO 4TH REAR OF R. LEG.—The body is a little forward, r. arm en couronne, l. arm in 2nd pos.

Exercise 13.   ARABESQUE OUVERTE.—L. leg 4th rear; bust inclined forward; r. arm stretched out forward; l. arm to rear; r. arm and l. leg forming a straight line; the body rests on r. foot.

Exercise 14.   ARABESQUE CROISÉE.—The same as last, the bust must not, however, incline forward so much.

Exercise 15. PIROUETTE ON THE COU-DE-PIED.—Position, 2nd plié, l. arm in 2nd, r. arm in 1st. Make a turn on the point of l.f., placing the point of the r. foot over the l. instep, the arms in repose.

Exercise 16. PIROUETTE À LA SECONDE EN L'AIR.—Position, same as the last, arms in 2nd. Turn on l.f. in making a battement in the 2nd with r.f.

Exercise 17. PIROUETTE ON THE POINT. In 5th foot position (fig. vi). In this place, rise on the points in 2nd (fig. 3), recover to 5th position in a single spring; then rising on the point of r.f., placing the point of l.f. over the instep and the arms en couronne, pirouette on the point of r.f.

Exercise 18. PREPARATION FOR THE PIROUETTE IN 4TH POSI-TION, feet in 4th position ; knees slightly bent ; right arm 1st position, l. arm 2nd position. In this position make a pirouette to the right, either on the instep or in the seconde or en arabesque or reversing ; throw l. arm forward touching the right, the two hands in 1st position, and make a turn to the right.

Exercise 19. PIROUETTE RENVERSÉE (Pirouette backward).— Position same as the last, only the bust inclined backward. In commencing the arms are en couronne and at the finish are in the 2nd position.

Exercise 20. THE 5TH ON THE POINTS. (Fig. VII). To arrive at this position. the feet must be flat in 5th position, and the arms in repose. **Bend** the knees lightly, then raise the heel with a little upward spring to rise on the points, the legs very straight, the arms en couronne ; then return to 5th ground position and repeat several times with either the right or left foot in front.

After having spent a considerable time in acquiring these preliminary positions and movements until they can be done with ease and aplomb, they may be practised rhythmically, that is, to music.

The principal study for the legs is to acquire a complete outward turn of the hips, knees and feet ; without this, grace is hopeless (See all the figures).

Pliés (bends, fig. viii.) may now be made in every position, great care being taken to *keep the heels on the floor.* Arms in 2nd position. Knees should be forced backward.

Study of the body. With the exception of certain attitudes and arabesques, *the body* should always be perpendicular (aplomb) and straight (droit) so as to throw the chest forward. *The head* should not remain fixed and immobile, but should slowly incline to one side according to which side the eyes are directed ; it must be kept high, countenance pleasant and expressive, shoulders down. The whole body must be firm and rest well but lightly on the hips which must never be agitated.

Centre of gravity. The dancer must always maintain the centre of gravity on the line of support, that is on the axis of the legs resting on the ground in the attitudes. In the arabesques, the centre of gravity is not so placed because the body bends forward, backward or to the side.

Simple position of the body (fig. i.)

Épaulement and opposition of the body (fig. iv. vi.)

Study of the Arms. The dancer must attach special importance to this branch of the art. It is the most difficult of all, and upon it chiefly depends the grace of the dance. The study may be divided into three parts, (1) positions, (2) opposition, (3) port de bras. Opposition is the contrast between the arms and feet.

The *elbow* and *wrist* must never be bent to form an angle, which is extremely ungraceful. They must be well-rounded with the arm (*arrondi*) so that the elbow and wrist become almost imperceptible in the general curve. Few dancers distinguish themselves in their arm movements, they imagine themselves perfect with a few brilliant movements of the legs— what a mistake! how much more brilliant would their dance appear with the appropriate graceful arm movements.

Arms in 2nd position (fig. i.)

Arms in opposition (fig. vi.)

Arms arrondi over the head en couronne (fig. vii.)

Demi-bras (fig. ii.)

Opposition of demi-bras (fig. iv.)

The student may now pass to the following practise:—

(1) GRANDS BATTEMENTS. Standing in 5th position, stretch out one leg horizontally (fig. ix.) and let it fall back again to the 5th position. These should be practised forward, backward and sideward.

(2) *Petits battements.*—The same as the last but the toe of the active foot does not leave the floor in passing from the 2nd to 5th position.

(3) *Petits battements sur le cou-de-pied* (on the instep).— The feet in 2nd position. The l.f. remains entirely on the ground and the point of r.f. only skims the ground in bringing either front or rear of the left with the heel raised and toes down.

RONDS DE JAMBE.—(1) *Rond de Jambes en dehors* (outward). The feet being in the 2nd position, the point of r.f. must, in gliding on the ground, describe a quarter-circle outward to the 4th rear, then bring to 1st position, carry it forward to 4th and make an outward half-circle to 4th rear; the l.f. must be steady.

(2) *Ronds de Jambe en dedans.*—The foot describes an inward circle; the inverse of the last exercise.

(3) *Rond de Jambe en l'air.*—The same as before, but while standing on one leg the other makes the circles in the air.

ENTRECHATS.—These are the most beautiful steps in dancing, if they are executed with grace and agility. They consist ot one or more rapid crossings of the feet while the dancer is in the air, then coming down in 5th position or some other attitude. The prettiest are the Entrechats à six and à six ouvert.

PIROUETTES require much and long hard practice. They consist of a turn in place on the point of the foot with perfect equilibrium. The dancer must have perfect aplomb before commencing a pirouette; he must place the arms in such a way as to acquire a force of propulsion in turning (as fig. viii. but with the r. arm brought across the chest) and at the end must step with aplomb and assurance.

DANSEUR SÉRIEUX, DANSEUR DEMI-CARACTÈRE, DANSEUR COMIQUE. Those who are destined for serious dancing must possess a good figure and pleasing form. The demi-caractère dancer must have an average figure, slim and elegant. The comic dancer must be vigourous and thick-set and have a moderate figure.

Among dancers there exist three classes:—

(1) The elegant and straight, with perfect limbs (fig. i.)

(2) The bow-legged, the inside of the legs forming a circle (see "bow-legs.")

(3) The knock-knee'd whose knees touch and the feet are open.

Thermestries.—Ancient Greek. With arms bare to the shoulder and handling long swords, the dancers run, attack one another, flee and return to the attack simulating victory and defeat.

Tire-Bouchon (pas) (TEER-BOO-SHAW), a corkscrew. Stretch the r. leg to 2nd elevation, the body turned to the left in such a manner that the r. heel points up and the toe down. Hop on l.f. at the same time, the r. leg pivots on the knee and hip describing a circle in the air while the body turns to the right, the r.f. will finish with toe pointing downward in the air. Put r.f. down, raise l.f. and repeat with other foot.

Tombé (pas) (TOMBAY) or RETOMBÉ. A fall. (*See* Sauté). After a spring, hop or jump (*saute*), there is naturally the alighting on one or both feet—this is tombé. The pas tombé is made by (1) bend both knees, (2) hop on r.f. and stretch l.f. to 2nd elevation, (3) cross l. leg rear of r. leg, drop on it and raise r. leg.

Tombé-Pointè.—After executing the preceding, finish by pointing the r. toe up with the heel on the ground, then assemblé. These movements with appropriate play of the arms make good comic steps.

Tom-Tit.—Bv Crompton, 1898. For one couple.

Tonadillas.—Very lively passionate Spanish dance of the Bolero type.

Tordion.—Old dance by Coquillart of Rheims, date 1450, in 3-4 tempo. It had some resemblance to a slow gaillarde and is mentioned as such in Feuillet's "Chorégraphie."

143

Tortillé (TAW-TEE-YAY).—Twisted, wreathed. A turning step to and tro in which it differs from tourné. It consists of two turns and is therefore a double or compound movement. Stand in 1st position. (1) Twist heel of r. foot outward, (2) put r. heel down and turn toe out, (3) turn toe in, down, (4) pivot r. sole and bring heel back to 1st position. It can also be made simultaneously with both feet.

Tour (TOOR).—A round movement whether executed in place or moving away from it. It is correct, therefore, to speak of a whole, half or quarter tour.

Tour de corps.—Turn of the body.

Tour en l'air (TOOR-AHN-LAIR).—Turn in the air. As the title suggests this is a complete turn, or several turns, during an upward spring off both feet, in the air. After bending both knees from 2nd position, spring upward vertically, turning while in the air, and alight on both feet assemblé or in attitude. To obtain this result, the student should first practice a quarter, then half, then three-quarter, finally a complete turn or more. The arms, before commencing, should be at the side opposite to that on which the turn is made. Example, to turn to the left; bend both knees and bring both arms outstretched to right side ready to swing them for the necessary momentum for the turn.

Tour des mains (TOOR DAY MEH).—Turn of the hands. Holding partner's hands while walking round in a circle. Thus also, *tour de main droite*, holding right hands; *tour de main gauche* holding left hands; *tour des deux mains*, holding the two hands. These movements are made facing each other.

Tourné (TOOR-NAY). Turning, A movement by which the whole leg is turned inward or outward. It is impossible to turn the foot without moving the rest of the leg. *Se tourner* is a turn of the body which can be done without any movement of the leg.

Tournure.—When presentiug a hand to partner, one naturally turns the body to look at the person, this is called *tournure.*

Tourniquet.—(*See* Moulinet).

Traktros.—Ancient Greek military dance.

Tragic Dances.—Greek dances were of three kinds:—Tragic, Comic and Satirical. The Tragic dances were noble, grave and majestic.

Traversé (TRAH-VER-SAY).—*See* Quadrille, fig. 2. To re-cross.

Trenchmore.—A popular dance in 6-4 tempo, in the sixteenth and seventeenth centuries. The earliest mention I find of it occurs in a Morality play by William Bulleyn in 1564, and the lastest in 1728. The figures and musical notes may be seen in the early editions of Playford's "Dancing Master" London, 1652. The directions there given for the dance are as follows:—

"Trenchmore; Longwayes for as many as will: Lead up all a D. (double) forwards and back three times, cast off, meet below, and come up, do so three times. First Cu. (couple) go down under the second Cu. (second couple's) arms, the three come up under the first; do this forward and back twice or thrice . . . . First man set to second W. (woman) then to his own, then to third W. then to his own, then to 4th W. then to his own, and so to all the W. (women) and men; then your W. do the same; then arm them as you set to them, arming your W. then your W. as much.

Lead up again, then turn your W. with your right hand and the 2nd with your left, your W. following as you turn till you come to your place, then your W. do the same, you following her, the rest doing these changes.

The music is a lively sixteen bars in six-eight time.

"Trenchmore" (the meaning of which we have to seek) was, however, more particularly the name of the dance than the tune. The dance, in fact, was performed to various tunes like our modern dances. In proof of this I quote from Taylor's "Navy of Land Ships," 1627. "Nimble-heel'd mariners (like so many dancers) capering in the pompes and vanities of this sinful world, sometimes a Morisco, or Trenchmore of forty miles long, to tune of "Dusty, my deare," "Dirty come thou to me," "Dun out of the mire," or "I waile in woe and plunge in paine;" all these dances have no other musicke."

In the Morality play by Bulleyn in 1564 is the following description of an old Minstrel. "Sir, there is lately come into this Hall, in a grene Kendale coat, with yellow hose, a bearde of the same colour onely upon the upper lippe: a russette hatte, with a great plume of straunge feathers and a brave scarfe about his necke in cut buskins. He is playing at the trea trippe with our host sonne; he plaieth tricke upon the gitterne (ancient musical instruments), and daunce Trenchmore and Hele de Gie and telleth news of Tera Florida."

Trenchmore is also mentioned in Stephen Gosson's "School of Abuse" (1579), and in Heywood's "A Woman killed with kindness" (1600). In "The Island Princess," by Beaumont and Fletcher, act v., one of the townsmen says "All the widows in the town dance a new Trench-more," and in the comedy of "The Rehearsal," the earth sun and moon are made to dance the Hey to the tune of Trenchmore. In part II. of Delaney's "History of the Gentle Craft" (1598) he says, "And in this case like one dancing Trenchmore, he stamped up and down the yard, holding his hips in his handes." Burton in his "Anatomy of Melancholy" (1621) says of Dancing, "Who can withstand it; be we young or old, though our teeth shake in our heads like Virginal Tacks, or stand parallel asunder like the arches of a bridge—there is no remedy; we must dance Trenchmore over tables chairs and stools.

145

The character of the dance as performed at that period may be gathered from this amusing quotation from Seldon's "Table Talk" (1689). "The Court of England is much altered. At a solemn dancing first you had the grave Measures, then the Corrantoes and Galliards, and this is kept up with Ceremony; at length the Trenchmore and the Cushion Dance, and then all the Company dance, Lord and Groom, Lady and Kitchen-maid, no distinction. So in our Court in Queen Elizabeth's time, Gravity and State were kept up. In King James's time things were pretty well, but in King Charles's time, there has been nothing but Trenchmore and Cushion Dance, omnium gatherum, tolly polly, hoite cum toite."

Trénis (SEE QUADRILLE, FIG. V.)

Trépignés (TEMPS). The dancer stands on the two heels, feet apart. In this way he advances, retires, or turns at his choice. The arms should be crossed in front or the hands on the hips.

Trévisane.—Italian dance, date 1752, 3—4 tempo quick. The couple hop twice on each foot, then giving right hands make a tour des mains and repeat with left hands, the step being the hop.

Trihori.—Ancient French dance, date 1589, mentioned by Arbeau. In 2—4 tempo. Three pas marches sideways or forward, then hop and assemblé. Rise (élevé) on l.f. then on r.f. and again on l.f.; repeat the pas marchés, hop and assemblé, and for the second time instead of élevés make a berceau. It was danced in groups of three dancers.

Triomphante.—Old French contredanse composed by Blasis. In the form of a quadrille the dancers performed some of the now well known figures of that dance.

Trot de Cheval, *pas* (TRO DER SHER-VAHL).—Horse trot. For Jigs, Hornpipes, Russian dances, etc. Hop on l.f. raising the r. knee forward bent, then pass r.f. rear of l.f. Repeat with other foot. To obtain the sound of the trotting horse is the object of the step. Thus, the foot resting on the ground, is, during the hop, beaten by the other foot. The step can be made forward, backward or in place.

Two-Step.—A modern dance but now almost obsolete. It was done to 2—4 tempo, by chassé forward, backward or turning.

Tyrolienne.—To music in 3—4 tempo. Partners stand side by side. Gentleman's r. hand holds lady's l. hand. Commence inside foot. Description of gentleman's step, lady does the counterpart.
Bar 1. (1) R.f. forward pas marché, (2) Repeat l.f., (3) Pause.
The weight of the body will be on rear foot. The arms should be carried forward and with the backs half-turned; look at each other.

Bar 2. (1) R.f. to 4th rear and dégagé, (2) L.f. to intermediate 3–4 position forward and arms to rear, (3) Pause.

Bars 3, 4, 5, 6. Polka, Polka Mazurka or Mazurka.

There are many Tyrolean dances usually accompanied by the "yodling" of the dancers but all are more or less alike.

V

Valaque.—Ancient Roumanian dance, date 1392. The couples formed in two parallel lines, men one line, women the other line. The dance was:—One step forward, one step back, turn to the right on the sole of one foot, repeat to left, then beat or lightly stamp while clapping hands in time, turning; they change places still beating hands and feet. Repeat ad lib.

Valse PAS DE.—(1) Glide r.f. forward, (2) glide l.f. forward, (3) r.f. to 3rd rear, (4) glide l.f. forward, (5) glide r.f. forward, (6) l.f. to 3rd rear. These take two bars and constitute *Pas de valse en avant,* or forward. For *pas de valse en arrière* or backward (1) l.f. to 4th rear, (2) r.f. to 4th rear, (3) l.f. to 3rd forward, (4) r.f. to 4th rear, (5) l.f. to 4th rear, (6) r.f. to 3rd forward (two bars). These movements are always done in a straight line forward or back. When the lady goes backward gentleman goes forward and vice versa, but the step is always the same, i.e., commence r.f. to go forward and l.f. to go backward. This step is also known as *Pas du Boston* and is the common Boston step forward or backward.

Valse (VAHLTZ) spelled also **Waltz.** It is claimed that Germany is the country of the origin of the Valse and the Germans call it their "genuine national dance." There is no doubt that the original Valse was "La Volte" which was sometimes called "Wolte." The German claim is refuted, and with good reason, by the French. Articles by Bouillet, Larousse and several Academicians appeared in "La Patrie" Paris on January 17th, 1882, and onwards, proving conclusively that the valse or volte was first danced in Paris, in 1178 or about 600 years before the Germans adopted it. That journal says "Scholars ruin the legend attributing to Germany the invention of the valse. The origin of the dance, which Murger calls "*le pas de charge de l'amour,*" is French. The valse did not take its birth in Germany, because from a description in a manuscript of the XIIth century, it was danced for the first time in Paris on the ninth of November, 1178. It was then already known in Provence as "la volte" and the chant which accompanied it was designated by the title "pallada." It came from Provence to Paris, became the mode during the XIIth century and was the delight of the Court of Valois. The Germans afterwards adopted it, and Provencal "volte" became the German "walzer." The music and dance are described as "en danse, un movement lent sur les deux premiers temps de la mesure, et en bref sur la troisième; en musique, deux notes, une blanche et une noire, font une mesure en trois temps." (*"For the dance, a slow movement on the first two beats of the measure, and a brief one for the third; for the music, two notes, one white and one black, making one measure in three time."*)

There are many forms of the valse, the most familiar are:— valse à deux temps, and valse à trois temps. Mention must also be made of "Hesitation Waltz" and "Boston" (which is variation of the pas de valse. The simplest form of the valse movement is "PAS DE VALSE, already mentioned. When dancing this with partners, gentleman should invariably go backward and lady forward. It can, however, be done *turning*:—Pivot a half-circle on counts 1 and 4 and make steps 2 and 5 sideways and assemblé to 3rd position on counts 3 and 6 this is the BOSTON step or PAS DU BOSTON.

Valse à deux pas.—(1) Glide l.f. to the side bending. (2) Glide r.f. to l.f. and chassé l.f. to side at the same time.

Valse à deux temps.—This is simply two hops on each foot in turning for every bar of 3-4 music.

. *Position.* In all Valses, the gentleman commences with his back to the centre and the lady faces the centre. The lady places her right hand fingers in the upturned palm of the gentleman's left hand, her left hand rests lightly on his upper right arm, while his lower right arm passes under her left arm and "enlaces" her with the hand at her back at the waist line. The gentleman's left elbow should be drawn in against his side.

Valse à l'envers (VAHLS AH LAHNVAY).—Valse Reverse. This is done by reversing the movements of the feet in the ordinary valse. It is, however, important that the movements are made in the same line of direction as the ordinary valse, and not the wrong way round the room. The gentleman begins with his back to the wall, then (1) r.f. to the right, (2) l.f. rear of r.f., (3) pivot on both soles now facing the wall, (4) l.f. forward between partner's two feet, (5) r.f. round, (6) l.f. between partner's two feet. This will complete a circle in two bars of music. The lady commences on the 4th step.

Valse à trois temps.—*The step* is composed of six temps occupying two bars of 3-4 music. *Lady's step:*—Position, facing centre of room. (1) Glide r.f. forward to 4th pos., between partner's feet, (2) pivot 1-6th of a circle on r. side and glide l.f. round to 2nd pos., (3) glide r.f. forward between partner's feet. These three steps during one bar of music will have completed one-half of the valse and formed a half-circle, finishing with the back to the centre of the room, (4) glide l.f. to the left, (5) keep weight on l.f. and glide r.f. to rear of l.f., (6) keeping the weight on l.f., pivot on both soles, finishing facing centre; this will take the second bar of music. The body of the dancer is turning the whole time, like a joint in front of the fire; it follows, therefore, that for a circle in six steps, the body must turn one-sixth circle for each step. Step 5 requires special care the weight of the body must be on l.f., and the sole of r.f. is placed in rear of l.f. as far back as possible *without disturbing the weight from l.f. or leaning backward* (it will be found that the space between the feet will be the length of one foot); the r.f. must not be too close to l.f. or the feet will catch in attempting to pivot for 6 and no pivot can be made. The gentleman commences with his back to the centre of the room and the steps are the same but in this order, 4, 5, 6, 1, 2, 3. Hence the combined lady's and gentleman's steps are:—1 and 4; 2 and 5; 3 and 6. The majority of dancers do not pivot on 6, but simply draw the l.f. to the r.f. Each dancer considers the partner as the centre round which he or she rotates, hence the r.f. which is nearest the centre must describe shorter steps whilst the l.f. which is farther must describe long steps. The movements must be done with elasticity ease and elegance. FOR REVERSE VALSE. The lady having simultaneously completed step 3 and gentleman step 6 of the valse, she will be with her back to the centre and he faces the centre; from this point the reverse is commenced thus:—

(1). Lady l.f. forward between partner's feet.
      Gentleman r.f. to side in 2nd position.

(2). Lady pivot 1-6th circle on l. sole and carry r.f. round to 2nd position.

      Gentleman carry l.f. to rear of r.f.

(3). Lady l.f. forward between partner's feet.
      Gentleman pivot on both soles.

The partners will now have changed their positions, and for counts 4, 5, 6, they exchange steps, that is, for count 4 the gentleman does lady's step 1, while she does gentleman's step 1, etc. The gentleman guiding, valses as many bars as he pleases to the right, reverse, forward or backward, the lady must easily follow his lead and she must carefully avoid throwing any undue weight on his supporting arm. What is known as a "heavy" dancer is due to two causes, first, taking short steps with l.f. and second, leaning heavily forward.

Valse Cotillon (COT-TEE-YON).—A square dance for 8 persons Stand as for ordinary square dances. The music is a slow valse. It is composed of six figures. When properly danced, this is perhaps the most beautiful of the square dances in vogue.

Figure 1.   1st couple waltz round the square once, occupying 16 bars.

Figure 2.   CHANGE OF PLACES.   The 1st and 2nd lady facing each other—(1, 2, 3,), balancé to right (4, 5, 6,), balancé to left (7 to 12), one valse movement to couple on the right with back turned to that couple: repeat this and finish in opposite places. This has taken 8 bars.

Side ladies repeat 8 bars.

Top gentlemen repeat 8 bars.

Side gentlemen repeat 8 bars; 32 bars. All will now be in opposite places.

Figure 3. 1st and 2nd couples valse to places (8 bars), side couples repeat (8 bars).

Figure 4. ALL VALSE CHAIN.—This is a simultaneous movement for all the dancers. Face partners and take right hands (1, 2, 3,), balancé forward r.f. (4, 5, 6,), balancé backward l.f. (7 to 12), one valse movement forward both commencing r.f. (4 bars in all). The gentlemen will now find themselves facing the lady on the right, and the ladies facing the gentleman on the left. (Unfortunately, this figure is seldom danced publicly in this way; the most common method is for the gentleman to seize the lady by both hands, and after a preliminary shake or two he twists her under his arms; if he isn't tall enough some ludicrous scene follows, sometimes disastrously to the lady's hair). *Care must be taken in the valse movement forward not to make an allemand or passing under the arm;* it is a simple forward valse. Repeat with next lady and again six times—eight times in all, *giving right hand each time.* After the eighth time, all will be in places. This figure occupies 32 bars.

Figure 5 VALSE PROMENADE ALL.—Join r. hands and l. hands crossed over the right. All with a gliding *pas marché* (walking step), one step to the bar, i.e., (counting 1, 2, 3, for each step), promenade round the square once to the right 16 steps. (16 bars).

Figure 6. GRAND VALSE ALL.—All valse round the square once to the right making eight valse movements during 16 bars.

Valse en cinque temps (VAHLS AHN SANK TAHM).—(Under the title "Half and Half," this dance was recently claimed by a New York teacher as his invention). In 1850 a Parisian dancing master published a dance composed of one measure of valse followed by a measure à deux temps. The dance is identical with the Half and Half and both movements are incorporated in one bar of 5-4 music. The step is composed of (counts 1, 2, 3,) a slow glide forward of l.f., (4) step forward r.f., (5) step forward l.f. For the next bar, reverse. The movement can be done forward, backward, turning, reverse, side by side and many variations. Note that the first step is commenced with alternate feet.

Valse Hesitation.—The principle of this dance is the pause on counts 2, 3, of the first bar in every valse movement. Thus:—

1, 2, 3, One bar { Gentleman pivot on l.f., describing half circle. Lady glide r.f. forward pivot, describing half circle.

4, 5, 6, One bar { Gentleman do second half of his valse movement completing the circle. Lady do second half of her valse movement completing the circle.

The steps can be made going forward or backward in a straight line.

Whether valsing forward or reversing, lady always takes step 1 with r.f., gentleman with l.f. Many variations may be introduced, the most common are "The Butterfly," the couples going alternately forward and backward, first the lady advances while he retires during a count of 6, then turning half-round she retires while he advances.

The step may be analysed as (1, 2, 3,) pas marché, glissade r.f., (4, 5, 6,) pas de valse, which can be done in any direction and varied at the taste of the dancer.

Valse Hesitation.—The Americans claim this dance as having emanated from New York in 1912, but an official description was published by l'Academie des Maitres de Danse de Paris many years before that. The Parisian description is as follows:—

It is composed of "pas de valse Boston" and "glissés." Position same as for "Boston." Tempo 3-4. Gentleman commences forward with right foot, lady backward with left foot.

(1), One "Pas de Valse Boston" turning a half-turn to the right (1 bar).

Glissé left foot en arrière for gentleman and the right foot en avant for the lady (1 bar).

During the glissé the free foot must be "pointé basse" (*pointed low*), and must be slowly drawn closer to the other foot during counts 2.3.).

"Pas de Valse Boston" en arrière with right foot for gentleman turning a half-turn to the left. Lady the same en avant (1 bar).

Glissé left foot en avant for gentleman, and right foot en arrière for lady (1 bar). These four bars are repeated *ad libitum*, but always the pas de Boston is made with the same foot—right foot for gentleman, left foot for lady.

(2). The steps just described are then made, keeping the lady at the side and making a half-turn on the "pas de Valse Boston," so as to follow always the same forward direction.

Description of change of position. At the commencement, the position is that of the Boston, and, during a Boston step, the gentleman makes the lady turn to the right a half-turn and takes her to his left side; his left arm will then be in front of her while the right is still about her waist (1 bar).

Glissé en arrière for gentleman and en avant for the lady, in this same position (1 bar), one pas de Valse Boston with half-turn to the left, which then places the lady "face en arrière" to the line of direction and the gentleman "face en avant," and the right arm of the lady finds itself in front of the gentleman. As before, these steps are repeated *ad lib.*

(3). LES PIVOTS. These pivots are made, one to each bar. The dancers may pivot twice, three or four times consecutively. To resume the dance it is necessary to make a "grand glissé (1 bar).

(4). " **The Back-Bend**" or " **Renversement en arrière.**"
This is perhaps the most graceful movement in the "Valse-Hesitation " and we specially draw attention to its close study.
Having made one movement of number 1 (1 bar) the
gentleman glissé left foot en arrière (1 bar), and instead of
withdrawing en arrière and turning to the left, he sets out en
avant with a pas de Valse Boston, making her " pivot " towards
the right. They then resume en avant or en arrière with
number 1 or 2. The pivot of the lady in the " renversement "
is simply the pas de Valse Boston, keeping the left foot almost
in place.

Many " fantasies " and variations may be introduced into
the Valse-Hesitation, but we advise dancers to preserve the
character and " chic " of the origin of the dance, and not abuse
them.

It will be observed that the Parisian description differs
from the American version in two important points; first, the
Parisian version makes the man always commence with r.f., in
the American version he begins with l.f.; second, the former
version makes the hesitation on bar 2. Nevertheless it will
be noticed that in both versions the Hesitation and Boston steps
are with the same feet, that is, gentleman always hesitates on
l.f., the lady on r.f., and gentleman commences pas de valse
with r.f., lady with l.f.

Varsovienne. (VAH-SO-VE-EN).—Round dance. Four bars of 3—4
music for 10 movements of the feet. Gentleman's step.

Part 1. (1) Glide l.f., (2) draw r.f. to l.f. and raise l.f.
to the side, (3) hop on r.f. and bring l.f. rear of r.f. (4, 5, 6,)
repeat 1, 2, 3, with same foot (2 bars).

Part 2. *Pas de Polka Varsovienne.* (7) Glide l.f., (8)
draw r.f. to l.f., (9) glide l.f. to the side (1 bar), (10) raise
and point r.f. to side and pose on that side, (11, 12,) retain
the pose (1 bar), repeat the four bars commencing with the
other foot. In the music there is a clear indication of the
pause and is sometimes written so that part 2 must first be
danced either four or eight times, followed by part 1 three
times, then part 2 once, but the music is an easy guide to the
parts which must be danced.

Veleta.—Modern round dance. 16 bars in 3—4 tempo. Partners
stand side by side, gentleman's r. hand holding lady's l. hand.
Description for gentlemen, ladies do counterpart.

Bar 1. (1, 2, 3,) Pas de valse forward l.f.

Bar 2. (4, 5, 6,) Repeat r.f. (finish facing partners and
take both hands).

Bar 3. (7, 8, 9,) Pas glissé to left, (7,) glide l.f. to left,
(8, 9,) draw r.f. to 3rd position with dégage.

Bar 4. (10, 11, 12,) Pas glissé to left, finish facing in
opposite direction and release r. hand.

4 *bars* (1—12). Repeat whole, commencing r.f. and in
retrograde direction, i.e., go forward, covering the previous

ground and finishing in the starting place. Then take partner as for an ordinary valse.

2 *bars* (1-6). One valse movement.

2 *bars* (7-12). Pas glissé to left, twice.

4 *bars* (1-12). Two valse movements. Repeat the whole *ad lib.*

Villanelle. By Desportes, 1580.—The word means "pastoral poetry" or "a dance tune." This dance was to music in 3-4 rhythm. It was rustic and gay in character and danced by the peasants (the word is derived from the Spanish "*vilano*," a peasant).

First part. A couple standing side by side (the lady at the right of the gentleman) without holding: they part, she with r.f. to the right, he with l.f. to the left. Lady's step:— Pliér (*bend*) l. leg, sauter (*hop*) on l.f. while raising the r. leg forward, pose r.f. on ground, chassé r.f. by the l.f., hop on r.f. crossing l.f. before r.f. the point touching the ground. Raise r.f. to rear, chassé l.f. by r.f. and assemblé. Repeat the whole.

Second Part. Glide l.f. forward, hop on l.f. while raising r.f. to rear, r.f. pas marché, l.f. pas marché, r.f. pas marché; glide l.f. forward, hop on it, raise r. foot to rear, point r.f. to side and bring back point of r.f. close to the point of l.f.

Virginia Reel.—(*See* Sir Roger de Coverley). It may surprise some to learn that no such gentleman as Roger de Coverley ever existed. The dance "Old Roger of Coverley for evermore; A Lancashire Hornpipe" is contained in Playford's "Dancing Master" (edition 1685). From this, Addison borrowed the name "Sir Roger de Coverley" for the articles in the "Spectator." The name Coverley is derived from Calverley a knight of Yorkshire whose family dates back to Richard I. The recent representative of the family, Sir Walter Calverley Trevelyan, communicated a note to this effect, and sent extracts from Ralph Thoresby's MS. account (1658), of the family of Calverley, of Calverley, Yorks. In the United States, the dance is known as "Virginia Reel," but in the State of Virginia it is danced and known as "My Aunt Margery"; in Scotland as "The Mantman comes on Monday."

Vis-à-Vis (VE-ZAH-VE). Opposite neighbour; in square dances, the persons facing each other. Example:—First lady or gentleman and either second lady or gentleman; also when partners are facing each other, they are standing *vis-à-vis* as distinguished from *dos-à-dos* which is back to back. (See *dos-à-dos*).

Vito, el. Andalusia speaks the final word in contrasts of the dance; for pure decorative beauty, variety of expression, intensive force, happy contrast of treatment, in short, in the art of the dance, who wishes more natural pantomime than is to be found in the dances of the Andalusian gipsies. *El Vito* and *Toreo Espanol* are extremely delicate in mimicry both narrating the bull-fight, the placing of *banderillas*, defence with the cape and final despatch of the bull. They combine strong movement with speed and grace.

Volta, Volte or Rivolta. (*See* Valse). The peasantry of Provence danced the Volte vigourously during the sixteenth century, but mention is made of it being danced in Paris in 1178. In the sixteenth century, it found great favour in France, required much dexterity and superseded the Basse dances. Arbeau's description shows its similarity to the waltz, but the original volte is hardly likely to be revived, for the gentleman made leaps and entrechats, lifting the lady high in the air as he turned round, so that she came down on the other side. The couple first made five steps to left, then five to the right. Then springing on l.f., r.f. raised, made a step forward, a wide spring, the feet uniting. Repeat with either foot, the couple turning all the time. In " Henry V." Shakespeare says " And teach La Voltas high, and swift Corantoes."

W

Waltz. (*See* Valse).

Waltz Cotillon. (*See* Valse Cotillon).

Waltz Menuet. A simple dance. The gentleman stands beside his partner with right arm round her waist, left hand on the hip; her left hand on his shoulder and the right hand hold the dress out. Both face forward. Gentleman commence l.f., lady r.f. Take four pas marchés, counting 3 for each step or one step to the bar (4 bars), followed by two ordinary waltz movements, holding partners in the usual manner (4 bars). Repeat *ad lib.*

Washington Post. A modern round dance, now obsolete.

Y

Yatagan. Dance of Turks and Arabs who perform it with naked sabres.

Z

Zapateado. Spanish Dance, 1820. Music 6-8 tempo. A noisy theatrical dance to castagnette accompaniment. The dancers face each other, then turning in place, they knock their heels together; they run across to change places going back to back (*dos-à-dos*), they stamp their feet turning, return to places beating their feet against each other.

Zéphir or Zephyr (PAS DE) also known as **Pas Tendu.** (*See* Tendu).

Zorongo. Spanish, 1841. Music 6-8 tempo. A couple, facing each other, clap their hands to the accompaniment of the music. First the couple beat each other's hands, then the man slaps the woman's hands, followed by the woman slapping the man's hands. Then "enlacing," they make pas marchés, to the right, to the left, forward, backward and turning.

Zulma. 1855, Oriental. Music 3-4 tempo.

THE END.

ERRATA.

P. 61.—"**Dessous**" *should be* under or to the rear.
„   "**Dessu**"   „   over or in front.

———— • ———— • ————

The oldest book on dancing is undoubtedly " L'acteur." (The Actor'). This is a description of the work which now lies before me :—

P. MICHAULT. Begins [folio 1, a] " L'ACTEUR.—Cy commence la danse des aveugles," (" Here commences the dance of the blind.") Ends [fol. 42 a]. Cy finist la danse des aveugles imprimee a a genesue." (" Here finishes the dance of the blind, printed in Geneva.") Printed in Geneva, 1480, 4-to. Black letter type. Four engravings in wood inclusive of that on the title-page representative of " L'acteur " and immediately following that word. 43 printed leaves: no signatures, catchwords or pagination. Printed in long lines in prose and verse, 24 lines to the full page.

P. MICHAULT. " La danse des aveugles moralisee. Nouellment imprimee a Paris." (" The moralised dance of the blind. Recently printed in Paris.") Paris, 4-to, 1501. Printed in long lines on 24 folios, 38 lines to a page.

" DANSE MACABRE," or Dance of Death. There are 114 editions in various European languages, dating from 1484 to 1892.

COPLAND, Robert. " Maner of Dauncing of base daunces after the use of France and other places." Translated out of French into English by Robert Copland. London 1521. This is apparently the earliest English work on the subject.

CORSO, da Rinaldo. " Dialogo del Ballo." Venetia 1558. 8-vo.

D'ESTREES, Jean. " Quatre livres de danseries." Paris 1564. 4-to.

NORTHBROOK, John. " A Treatise wherein, Dicing, Dauncing, Vain Plaies, or Enterludes, with other pastimes, etc., commonly used on Sabbath Daies are by the Word of God reproved.' London 1579.

" THE DOLEFUL DANCE and Song of Death; intituled Dance after my pipe." 1577.

FETHERSTONE, Christopher. " A dialogue against light, lewde, and lasciuious Dauncing wherein are refuted all those reasons which the common people bring in defence thereof.", London 1582. 8-vo.

BEAUJOYEULX. "Ballet comique de la rogue." Paris 1582. 4-to.

(Same Author) "Ballets representez a Tours." Paris 1593. 4-to.

(Same Author) "Recueil de plusieurs excellents ballets de ce temps." Paris 1612.

(Same Author) "Discours au vray du ballet danse par le roy." Paris 1617. 4-to.

(Same Author) "Relation du grand ballet du roy de France en le salle du Louvre en 1619. Paris. 8-vo.

CAROSO (da Sermoneta) "Il Ballarino," with numerous plates by Giacomo Francho, of figures dancing in elegant Venetian costumes. Venice 1581.

ARBEAU, Thoinet. A monk who assumed the non de plume of "Tarburot." "Orchesographie: traite pour apprendre et pratiquer l'honnete exercise des danses." Langres 1588. 4-to. (This book is undoubtedly the first work pourtraying dances by dance alphabet figures.)

LOVELL, Thomas. "A dialogue between Custome and Veritie, concerning the use and abuse of Dauncing and Minstrelsie," (in verse) London, no date but probably about 1590. 8-vo.

DAVIES, Sir John (Attorney-Gen. of Ireland). "Hymns of Astrea, whereunto is added Orchestra, or a poem of Dauncing in a Dialogue between Penelope and one of her wooers " (not finished) 1596.

NEGRI, Cesare. "La Gratie d'Amore, detto il Trombone." Milan 1602, small folio.

(Same Author). "Nuove inventioni di Balli, opera vaghissima di Cesare Negri Milanese detto il Trombone, famoso et excellente Professore di Ballare." Milan 1604. (Small folio with portrait within an ornamental border and 58 engraved plates of Dancers by Leon Palavacino and with the music of the dances.

SARAZIN. "Recueil des masquerades et jeux de prix a la course du Sarazin fait ce keresme-prenant en le presence de sa majeste." Paris 1607. 12-mo.

(Same Author) "Recueil des plus excellentes ballets de ce temps. Paris 1612. 8-vo.

ROSCIO, J. L. "Brief conclusion of Dancing and Dancers." London 1609. 4-to.

EYORDIUS, James, of Helmstadt. A Treatise "de Saltationibus Neterum." Leyden 1611.

BORDIER. "Le Ballet du Hazard." Paris 1622. 8-vo.

BROWN, (or Browne) Richard. "Medica Musica, or a Mechanical Essay on the effects of singing Music or Dancing on Human Bodies," London 1624. 8-vo.

SICOGNES. "Le Ballet danse a Fontaine-Blue par des dames d'amour." Paris 1625. 8-vo.

(Same Author) "Le Ballet des Quolibets." Paris 1627. 8-vo.

(Same Author) "Le Ballet des Andovilles, porte en guise de Momen." London 1628. 8-vo.

PLAYFORD, John. "DANCING MASTER," or plaine and easy rules for the dancing of Country Dancing, with the tune to each Dance." London 1652. Oblong 12-mo. 17 editions, last edition published 1721.

"DANCING MASTER." Vol. 2, published 1728.

The Same. Vol. 3, published 1729.

BENTHAM, Joseph. "Treatise on the nature and accidents of mixed Dancing." London 1657.

WYCHERLEY, Wm. "The Gentleman Dancing Master." A Comedy. London 1673.

ANONYMOUS. "Les Plaisirs de l'isle Enchantée." Paris 1673, in folio.

MENESTRIER, P. "Des ballets anciens et modernes." Paris 1682. 4-to.

TUCCARO. "Trois dialogue de l'exercise de sauter et voltiger." Paris 1599. 4-to.

FEUILLET. "Recueil de Contredanses mises en Chorégraphie" par Mons. Feuillet, Maitre et Compositeur de Danse. Paris 1706. 12-mo. 109 leaves entirely engraved, containing title, dedication, preface, Élements de Choregraphie, instructions for the figures, etc., in 16 unnumbered leaves, followed by the music of each dance and the delineation of the figures in 186 numbered pages. Old calf. An extremely rare work and of great importance in its class, yet unknown and undescribed by the bibliographers. The Author admits in his preface the English were the inventors of the Contredanse and many of the airs contained in the book are English.

(Same Author) "Orchesography, or the Art of Dancing by Characters and Demonstrative Figures." Translated by John Weaver, Dancing Master. "To this edition is added the Rigadoon, the Louver and the Brittaigne in Characters . . . The whole engraven and printed for John Walsh in London 1700." (The music of the additional dances is given). See Weaver, John.

(Same Author) "La Choregraphie, ou l'art de decrue la danse." Paris 1713. 4-to. (The Author was assisted in this work by Desais).

WEAVER, John. "Art of Dancing by Characters and Demonstrative Figures." London 1706. 4-to.

(Same Author) " Essay towards an History on Dancing, in which the whole Art and its various Excellencies are in some manner explained." London 1712. 8-vo.

(Same Author,) "Anatomical and Mechanical Lectures on Dancing." London 1712.

ESSEX, John. "A Treatise on Dancing Country Dances." London 1710. 8-vo.

PEMBERTON, E. " An Essay for the further improvement of Dancing, being a collection of Figure Dances, of several numbers, composed by the most eminent masters: described in characters after the newest manner of Monsieur Feuillet." (Very scarce). London 1711. 4-to. It contains title, dedication, to Mr. Caverley, another to " The Duchess of Buckingham and Normandy," preface, list of subscribers (5 leaves) and 54 engraved leaves giving the notation of the dances and music.

MELETAON. " On the Excellencies of Dancing." (In German). Leipzig 1713.

LAMBRANZI. " Nuova e Curiosa Scuola de Balli Theatrali, continente cinpuanta Balli, di diverse nationi, e figure Theatrali, con i loro Vestimenti, etc. Inuentati e dati alla luce da Gregorio Lambranzi, Maestro de Balli Francesi . . .disegrati e intagliati da G. G. Cuschner." 2 parts or vols. In one small folio, consisting of 101 copper plate engravings of Dances with Music; fine copy, red morocco extra, profusely gilt by De Coverley. Nuremburg 1716. A copy of this work was recently on sale by Tauschnitz (price £75). It is very rare, and consists of Frontispiece on which is engraved portrait of the Author and the words " Deliceae Theatrales," prefatory note by the author in Italian and German, and description of the plates in Italian, 2 leaves, title as above engraved—" Sarte prima " 50 plates: " Zweiter Theil," title (engraved) and 51 plates. The plates represent burlesque figures and dances and have the music at the top, and the descriptions (in German) at the foot, all engraved. The second part is excessively rare.

TAUBERT, GOTTFRIED. " The History, Ethics, Theory, Practice and Composition of Dances." (German). Leipzig 1717.

LANDRIN. " Recueil de Musique, Contre-danses, les plaisirs de Mendon, etc." 70 feuilles of Dances with music. Paris 1720.

BONNET. " Histoire de la Danse." Paris 1724. 12-mo calf.

JENYNS, Soame. An elegant and ingenious writer (born in London 1703, died 1787). " Art of Dancing," A Poem. London 1730.

BURETTE, Peter John. A very celebrated musician, born Paris 1665, died 1747. He had a very considerable share in publishing the " Journal des Scravans " in 1706, at which he laboured more than 30 years. He also supplied the Memoirs of the Academie des Inscrip. et Belles Lettres with " Dissertations on the Dancing of the Ancients," and enriched these with music notes and remarks.

TOMLINSON, K. "Art of Dancing explained by reading and figures." London 1735. 4-to.

ANONYMOUS. "XII. Englische Taentzin mit Touren fur 2 Violin, 2 Flauten, 2 Waldhorn und Bass." Printed Neuwied 1740. 32-mo. 12 cards each with figures of a dance and engraving above, and 12 other cards with the tunes engraved, in the original paper case; probably unique.

FERRIOL OF BOXERAUS. D.de. "Reglas Utiles para los aficionados a Danzar provechose divertimiento de los que gustan instrumentos." Contains very curious woodcuts with folding leaves of music, some defective. Printed on vellum Capua 1745. 12-mo.

RAMEAU. "Le Maitre a Danser." Frontispiece and numerous engravings and plates. Paris 1748. Calf 8-vo.

OWEN. "Characters in Dancing drawn from real life." London 1749.

LANG, Karl. "The foundation of Dancing." (German). Palm 1751.

(Same Author) "Choreographic signs of the English and French Contre-danses." Palm 1763.

FONTAINEBLEAU. "La Danse, Acte de Ballet." (In verse). "Spectacles donnes a Fontainebleau." Vol. 1. 1753. 4-to.

CAHUSAC. "La danse ancienne et moderne, ou traite de la danse." 3 vols. Printed at the Hague 1754. 12-mo. See note to Gallini 1762.

"The Dancers Damm'd; or the devil to pay at the old house." London 1755. 8-vo.

MEREAU. "Reflexions sur le Maintien et sur les Moyen d'en corriger les Defauts." Gotha 1760.

CUISSE, de la. "Le repertoire des bals ou théorie practique des contre-danses descrites d'une maniere aisee, avec des figures demonstratives pour les pouvoir danser facilement, auxquelles on a ajoute les aires notes par le Signor de la Cuisse, Maitre de dause." Paris 1762-65. 4-to.

GALLINI, Sir John, (or as he styles himself in his Treatise Giovanni Andrea Gallini) a native of Italy and celebrated stage dancer and teacher of Dancing; died in London, where he long resided, 1805, aged about 71. "A Treatise on the Art on Dancing." London 1762, 1765, 1772. 2 vols. *This Treatise was very popular for some time, even as a literary performance, until, unluckily for Sir John, all the historical part of his publication was discovered in the work of M. Cahusac. See Cahusac.*

(Same Author) "Critical observations on the Art of Dancing with Music of 50 French Dances. London 1762.

(Same Author) "Treatise on the Art of Dancing." London 1762. (*Both books were published in* 1 *vol.* 8-*vo. calf at* 7*s.* 6*d.*)

THOMPSON. "Compleat collection of 200 Favourite Country Dances, performed at Court, Bath, Tunbridge, and all Publick Assemblies, with proper figures or directions to each Tune. (*Very scarce*). 3 vols. oblong 8-vo. (the third vol. deficient in leaves 52, 53, 54,) with ms. notes by Mr. Chappell. London 1765-1775.

SCHROEDER. "Dance-craft; to dance Choreographically and to write dances. (*German*). Brunswick 1767.

SCHULTZ, Barth. "Twelve new English Dances." (*German*). Hamburg 1783.

MARTINET. "Theory of Dancing." (*German*). Liepsig 1798.

ANONYMOUS. "Dancing Maskiana: or Biographic Sketches for an Inquisitive Public; being the true style of a Dancing Master, exhibiting his pupils at an Elegant Ball." London 1799. 8-vo. (pub. at 4/-).

MAGRI, G. "Trattato teorico-practico di ballo." Illustrated. Naples 1799. 2 vols. 4-to.

GRETRI. (A.E.M.) Melee de Chants et de Danses. Paris 1771. 8-vo.

POCKET COMPANION for the Guitar containing XI. of the newest and most favourite Minuets, Country Dances, etc. London, no date, but 18th Century.

CORELLI (Archangelo). Preludii Allemande, correnti, gighe, sarabande, gavotte e follia. London 1700. Oblong 4-to.

COMPLEAT COUNTRY DANCING MASTER, containing a great variety of Dances both old and new; particularly those performed at the several Masquerades with their proper tunes and figures to each dance. 2 vols. London 1718. 8-vo.

MAGNY. Princepes de Choregraphie. Paris 1765.

FISHAR, (James). 16 Cotillons, 16 Minuets, 12 Allemands and 12 Hornpipes. London 1775. 4-to.

PRESTON. Country Dances. London 1797.

ORCHESTIKOS, G. "Convivialia et Saltatona; or a few thoughts on Dancing and Feasting; a poem in two parts: to which is annexed a poetical epistle in praise of Tobacco." London 1800.

NOVERRE. "Lettres sur la Danse, sur les Ballets et les Arts." Par M. Noverre ancien maitre des ballets en chef de la Cour de Vienne et de l'Opera de Paris. With portrait. St. Petersburg, 1803. 4-to.

The third volume is entitled "Observations sur la construction d'une salle d'opera et programmes des Ballets.

WARES, (G. Junr.) Sketches and Observations on the necessity of early tuition in the Art of Dancing. London 1805. 8-vo.

PEACOCK, (Francis). "Sketches relative to the History and Theory, but more especially the Practice of Dancing." Aberdeen 1808. 8-vo.

WILSON, (Th). "Analysis of Country Dancing." London 1809. 8-vo.

(Same). "The Treasures of Terpsichore," or a Companion for the Ballroom. London 1809. 8-vo.

(Same). "Correct method of Waltzing the truly fashionable species of Dancing French and German Waltzing." Contains frontispiece, plates and music. London 1816. 12-mo.

(Same). "Companion to the Ballroom, a collection of Country Dances, Reels, Hornpipes, Waltzes, etc." London 1820. 12-mo. with music.

(Same). "Complete system of English Country Dancing." Engraved diagrams and examples of music. London 1828. 12-mo.

ANONYMOUS. "The Dance of Life." A Poem. London 1817. 8-vo.

DANCE. "Le maitre a danser, or the Art of Dancing Quadrilles." London 1818. 12-mo.

BARON. "Lettres et entreatiens sur la danse ancienne, moderne, religieuse, civile et theatrale." Paris 1824. 8-vo.

IZTUETA (J. E. Ignatio). "Guipuzcoaco Dantza." San Sebastian 1824. 8-vo.

ANONYMOUS. "Quadrille de Marie Stuart." Paris 1829. Small folio.

BLASIS (Carlo). "Art of Dancing, its theory, practice, rise and progress." Containing frontispiece and 17 engraved plates of numerous figures, and 22 pages of Quadrille music. London 1830. 8-vo.

(Same). "Notes upon Dancing, historical and practical." London 1847. 8-vo.

KELLY (Earl of). "Minuets." Edited with introduction by C. K. Sharpe, portrait and engraved title. Edinburgh 1836. 4-to. Only 60 copies were printed.

ANONYMOUS. "An Essay on the Art of Dancing viewed in connection with physical education." London 1838. 8-vo.

COKE-SMYTH. "Souvenir of the Ball costume given by Queen Victoria at Buckingham Palace with description by Planche." London 1842. In folio.

LAFAGE, (A. de). "Histoire Generale de la Musique et de la Danse." Contains music and 28 *fac-similes* and plates of instruments and dance figures. Two volumes. Paris 1844. 4-to.

FROM 1837 TO 1855.

CELLARIUS. "Drawing Room Dances."

(Same Author). "Fashionable Dancing."

COULON. "Handbook of Dancing."

READ. "National Dances."

HENDERSON. "New and fashionable Guide of Dances."

WEBSTER. "Dancing a means of Physical Education."

HART. "Dancing Art, its defence."

MASON. "Dancing considered."

DUNS. "Manual of Dancing."

KNOX (A. E.) "Spirit of the Polka."

ANONYMOUS. "Polka and Ballromm Guide." How to dance the Polka. Polka Lesson Book.

SAINT-LEON. "Stenochorographie." Moyen de fixer par des signes positifs tous les mouvements et tous les enchainements d'un opera. Paris 1852. In folio.

MODERN PERIOD.

FORFAR (W. B.) "Hilston Furry Day." Its origin, celebration and Music of the Furry Dance. London 1861.

THELEAUX (E. A.) "Letters on Dancing."

COOTE. "Dancing without a master."

HILL GROVE, (New York). "Complete guide to the Art of Dancing."

ANONYMOUS. "Danse du Monde and Quadrille preceptor."

DODWORTH. "Dancing, its relation to education."

ANONYMOUS. "Dancing in a Right Spirit a Delightful and Scriptural Pleasure." 1865. 32-mo.

ANONYMOUS. "Les Danses et les Bals d'aujourdhui, la lecture des romans, et les spectacles au point de vue moral et Chretien." Le Mans 1863. 12-mo.

ANONYMOUS. "The Dance, may I not join it ? or the Christian professor in the Ballroom." Ipswich 1864. 16-mo.

ANONYMOUS. "The Dance at the Feast and what came of it." London 1868.

ANONYMOUS. "Etiquette, How to Dance." London 1876. 32-mo.

HENDERSON (Mrs. N.) "Etiquette of the Ballroom." London 1879. 32-mo.

SAUSE (M. J.) "The Art of Dancing." New York 1880. 16-mo.

COOTE (R.) "Guide to Ballroom Dancing, etc." London 1876. 32-mo.

GROSS (J. B.) "The Parson on Dancing." Philadelphia 1879. 8-vo.

WALLACE (J. F.) "Excelsior Manual of Dancing." Glasgow 1881. 12-mo.

LEBLANC (Edw.) "Companion to the Ballroom." London 1883. 16-mo.

BOEHME (F. M.) "Geschichte des Tanzes in Deutchland.' Liepzig 1886. 8-vo.

STEELE (L.) "Drawing Room Dancing." Ealing 1883. 16-mo.

FLACH (H. L. M.) "Der Tanz bei den Griechen." Virchow 1880.

DONALDSON (H.) "Dancing, is it a sin?" Oil City, Pa., 1881. 8-vo.

QUELLIEN (N.) "Chansons et Danses des Bretons." pp. 300. Paris 1889. 8-vo.

HUMPHREY (E.) "London Ballroom Guide." pp. 89. London 1889. 32-mo.

MARRIOT (A.) "Dancing as an Art." pp. 67. Nottingham 1888. 16-mo.

MIGNON (P.) "Les Quadrille des variétés françaises." Paris 1883 Obl. 4-to.

PENTECOST (G. F.) "The Christian and the modern dance." pp.62. London 1884. 16-mo.

SCOTT (Edw.) "Dancing as it should be." London 1887. 16-mo.

ZORN (F. A.) "Grammatik der Tanzkunst." pp. 275. Leipzig 1887. 8-vo.

VESTRIS (D.) "Les danses d'autrefois." 120 pp. Paris 1889. 8-vo.

BERNAY (B.) "La danse au Theatre." 194 pp. Paris 1890. 8-vo.

ROWE (W. W.) "Dancing as it is." 22 pp. London 1890. 12-mo.

DUNALDOR (J.) "La Danse." pp. 118. St. Amand 1894 8-vo.

GIRAUDET (E.) "Traité de la Danse." pp. 287. Paris 1891. 8-vo.

GROVE (L.) "Dancing." (Badminton Library). pp. 496. London 1895. 4-to.

HEADLAM (S. D.) "The Ballet." pp. 16. London 1894. 8-vo.

HOGAN (J. P.) "Method of Dancing." New York 1892. 4-to.

HOW. "How to Dance." pp. 49. London 1893. 4-to.

IMAGE (S.) "The Art of Dancing." pp. 20. London 1891. 8-vo.

d'ALBERT (Charles). "Encyclopaedia and Technical Glossary of the Art of Dancing." London 1914-1915. 8-vo.

Lightning Source UK Ltd.
Milton Keynes UK
UKOW05f1824241013

219739UK00001B/24/P

9 781906 830595